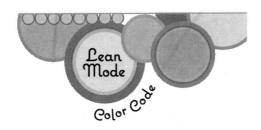

# Not Your Usual Food Diary

From the creators of the popular Streaming Colors™ Fitness Journal "healthy habit-forming calendar", comes the new Lean Mode, Color Code—Not Your Usual Food Diary, with PowerCircles™ and FoodDots™ to color in and connect, and a full page to record each day's details. Jen and Alexis Luhrs, mom/daughter publishing/creative team behind ColorCode Mode™ Journals, have had a lifelong devotion to healthy eating habits and preventive health, formalized when Jen worked with the Stanford Prevention Research Center in 1996 as writer/creative director on the HealthBuzz™ health improvement web site that was co-branded with msnbc.com. Trained in Industrial Design (Jen) and Architecture (Alexis), both women strive to create health improvement tools that are visually intuitive and adaptable, grounded in established principles of health behavior change, and most of all—easy and fun to use.

### Other ColorCode Mode™ Journals from Jen and Alexis Luhrs:

Streaming Colors™ Fitness Journal Weekly Planner – School Year (NEW in Sept. 2008)

Streaming Colors™ Fitness Journal Weekly Planner (since 2008)

Streaming Colors™ Fitness Journal Monthly Calendar (since 2004)

"Who hasn't heard the advice (at least once) to keep a diet journal? If you haven't tried it, here's one more reason to: a recent Centers for Disease Control study shows people who lose weight and keep it off use some system to track their progress....Little successes—like how many servings of veggies you eat or the number of tempting treats you manage to pass up—are all worth a note in your log....Our pick: the Streaming Colors Fitness Journal."

—**HEALTH magazine**, "Count Off the Pounds: Tools to Track Your Way to a Slimmer Body"

"Fit In Some Organization—Having trouble sticking with that New Year's resolution? Scheduling your workouts will increase your chances of staying on track...Streaming Colors workout calendar is a planner using color-coded markers to turn your sweat sessions into a work of art..."

—**FITNESS magazine**, "Fit Forecast"

Color yourself fit. The concept is similar to getting a gold star from the teacher for a job well done."

—**OXYGEN magazine**

Learn more at www.colorcodemode.com

CHARTER EDITION

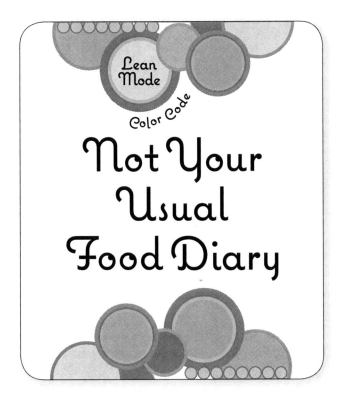

Lean Mode

Color Code

# Not Your Usual Food Diary

A **ColorCode Mode**™ Journal

Jen & Alexis Luhrs

HALF YEAR DIARY

LUHRS MEDIA CO.

Lean Mode, Color Code™, PowerCircles™, Connect-the-FoodDots™, ColorCode Mode™ and Not Your Usual Food Diary™ are trademarks of Luhrs Media Co.

Lean Mode, Color Code™ Food Diaries may be purchased and/or customized for educational, business, or sales promotional use. Contact the publisher at the above address, or at sales@colorcodemode.com.

Charter Edition

Design Concept and Content by Jennifer Luhrs and Alexis Luhrs

Graphic Design by Carolyn Gilde

Printed on acid-free, archival quality paper. **To avoid ink bleed-through, use highlighting pens, not markers.**

ISBN-10: 0-9821406-0-6
ISBN-13: 978-0-9821406-0-4

Nothing in this food diary/journal is intended as a substitute for medical advice or counseling. Consult your doctor if you have any risk factor or health-related condition that might prevent you from using this food diary/journal as a fitness tool. This food diary/journal is intended as a health promotion tool, not as a medical or physical therapy intervention. Luhrs Media Co. makes no claims whatsoever regarding the utilization or interpretation of any information contained herein and/or recorded by the user in this food diary/journal. Designed for adults and older teens in normal health. Not designed for unsupervised use by children. We are developing products for the special needs of children.

www.colorcodemode.com

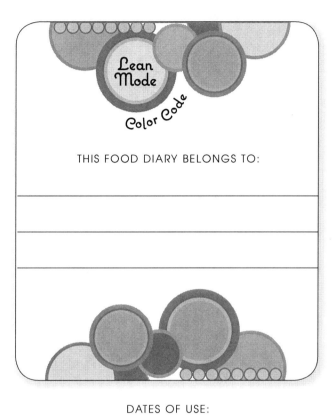

**Lean Mode**

*Color Code*

THIS FOOD DIARY BELONGS TO:

_____

_____

DATES OF USE:

_____ THRU _____

# Contents

# I.    Not Your Usual Food Diary Intro

How do you lose weight and keep it off if you keep going back to all your usual places and eating all your usual foods, in all your usual quantities? No wonder your last diet tanked. You're still slave to all your usual habits, those stubborn little backseat drivers of your lifestyle.

You need to do something unusual to tweak, nudge or cajole your eating and exercise habits into better shape.

Switch into Lean Mode and put your naughty, lazy habits on notice that things are going to change, and you have the proven tool to do it. Studies show that keeping a food diary is the key to successful long-term weight loss, including LOSING TWICE AS MUCH WEIGHT as those who don't journal.

If your habits aren't exactly shaking in their boots, maybe it's because they don't believe you'll stick with something as dry as writing in a food diary every day. See how well they know you?

That's why the Lean Mode, Color Code Food Diary was created to be anything but your usual food diary. In Lean Mode you'll use color-coding to round up all your usual bad habits and get them out into the open where you can keep a sharp, steady eye on them.

Not only will color coding help you spot trends—coloring is fun! It can reward you for making better choices, such as adding veggies or having a candy-bar-free day. It's been known to motivate people up off the couch to exercise so they'll have something to color in—not just another empty white day. It's faster and easier than writing (there's room for that, too) and entices you to make entering something positive in your diary your "usual" daily habit—which is very much the point.

Physical changes usually take time. Seeing a lot of color in your journal will help you feel more accomplished even if your body isn't yet showing results. Looking back over time at all that color will remind you of your ability to keep making positive changes.

The Lean Mode Food Diary comes with just two rules, and leaves everything else up to you, like what to change and when to change (after all, they're your bad habits), goals, rewards, how much detail, and (of course) which colors to use!

## RULE #1: COLOR IN ONLY THE GOOD THINGS YOU DO.

You're trying to reward positive actions in order to repeat them often enough to crowd out your usual crummy habits.

## RULE #2: COLOR IN SOMETHING EVERY DAY.

Consistency and small steps are the key to establishing healthy habits and losing more weight.

You could hold out for massive doses of willpower to magically appear and transform your bad habits for you. Or, you could try coloring in the FoodDots and PowerCircles of your Lean Mode Food Diary. After time, your habits will still be running you around, because that's what habits usually do. Only now you'll be running with a much better crowd.

"Habit is either the best of servants or the worst of masters."

*Nathaniel Emmons*
*(1745 - 1840)*

"Nothing is stronger than habit."

*Ovid*
*(43 B.C. - 17 A.D.)*

## II.    Some People —

## Why 21st Century People Need Food Diaries (and People 50 Years Ago Didn't)

SOME PEOPLE ARE JUST NATURALLY SKINNY.

With metabolisms that rival blast furnaces these people can eat all they want and never gain weight. That's probably not you if you're reading this book.

MANY PEOPLE TODAY BELIEVE THEY'RE DOOMED TO BE OVERWEIGHT —

unless they're willing to feel miserable and deprived. Is it any wonder? Everywhere you go, fast food drive-thrus beckon. The packaged food aisles in our grocery stores reel us in like kids in a candy store. Well meaning but sabotaging friends, family and co-workers ply us with high calorie foods and snacks. Now kids are learning their formative eating habits from a generation of young parents who think french fries and soda pop are two of the major food groups.

Obesity rates are soaring but few are willing to leave the party. How did we get into this super-sized, over-salted, deep-fried downward spiral?

MOST PEOPLE IN 1950'S AMERICA WERE NATURALLY THIN BY TODAY'S STANDARDS.

(And the few that weren't may actually have had the "fat genes" so many of us today blame for our "fat jeans.")

1950'S PEOPLE WEREN'T POSSESSED OF A SPECIAL WILLPOWER.

They were less informed about food and health risks than we are. And they didn't support a $35 billion dollar a year weight loss industry.

What was their secret to being able to fit into real size 8's, before the invention of Spandex in 1959— and long before the clothing industry made size 8's a lot bigger so we wouldn't all feel so bad?

The answer has nothing to do with willpower. 50's folks were just doing what came naturally in their popular culture. With the food and transportation systems of the time, 1950's people were simply in the HABIT of eating fewer calories and getting more physical activity than we do today.

They didn't feel particularly deprived or know what they were missing. They felt modern and happy to have flashy tailfin cars. But two-car households were rare—which means people often walked places, and most kids walked to and from school.

A typical household might be fortunate to have one TV, but it would be two decades or more before home computers, video games and TV's all over the house turned us into a nation of sit-all-day compulsive screen viewers and kids who rarely play outside.

In the 50's there was penny candy and an occasional trip to the root beer stand, but junk foods and fast foods weren't in peoples' faces 24/7. Gas stations weren't 24-hour junk food stations that also sold gas. In 1955, our popular culture hadn't yet been "super-sized." There were only 9 McDonald's in all of America. Today McDonald's feeds 47 million people worldwide EVERY DAY. And that's just McDonald's.

In the 1950's, most people ate most of their meals at home, and most of those meals were simple, home-cooked foods in reasonable portions (families were larger so food had to be divvied up between more people.) Between meals, people might experience a sensation called hunger, and without junk foods or fast foods at their fingertips, they probably burned off some body fat waiting for the next sit-down meal.

Lucky ducks, those 50's people—to not be faced with the constant temptations we're faced with every day. Somewhere along the way, we reached a tipping point where we had just too much of everything.

Now, *we know* — we can't turn back the clock, but we do have something in common with those blissfully unaware lean people of the 1950's. It's the same thing we have in common with every generation of humans. It's our habits—and we can harness them to create a personal comfort zone where we can become healthy and fit without feeling deprived.

## ALL PEOPLE ARE CREATURES OF HABIT.

Habits make daily life easier, because they are so mindless. Like brushing your teeth in the morning, they don't entail agonizing choices or decisions, or feelings of deprivation. 1950's people ate fewer calories and were more active than us because their environment and popular culture just naturally steered them into those habits.

Never underestimate the power of the seemingly innocuous little 5-letter word "habit." Habits play a role in our very survival. Instead of getting up in the morning and drinking antifreeze and eating gravel, we automatically, for example, have a cup of java and some toast. We don't overthink the decision, because hey, it's just a habit—something we've learned by repeating a behavior over and over.

Chances are our parents got us started on our food habits, and that's why the thought of having hissing Madagascar cockroaches for breakfast, for example, just doesn't cross our minds.

If all of your habits are healthy, yay for you because they'll make it easy for you to sustain the healthy lifestyle all the experts keep telling us we should have. That lifestyle is made up of the accumulation of habits we repeat every day.

If you're reading this book because some (or most!) of your habits are unhealthy, and you want to change them, you're going to need the help offered here. That's because habits have an ironic flip side. They're mindless when in place, but to

change them, you have to be quite mindful, at least for a while.

Yes, your habits are stubborn little buggers when it comes to being changed. Experts say it takes about 30 days of repeatedly practicing a behavior for it to become an established new habit. But we think it takes longer with eating habits. The temptations to backslide are strong given the prevalence of junk foods and the many distractions of today's popular culture.

Even with TV, those lucky 1950's people were exposed to only the tip of the advertising and marketing iceberg that keeps sinking our attempts today to stay focused on healthier habits. Here's why it's so much harder for us today:

## MARKETING PEOPLE USE POWERFUL TOOLS TO ENTICE YOU TO MAKE THEIR PRODUCTS A HABIT.

Marketers aren't inherently bad people (we know because we're marketers ourselves.) But a marketer's job is to get you to repeatedly buy a product regardless of whether it's good for you or not.

From media campaigns and fast-food restaurant locations and signage, to shelf location that puts brightly colored overly-packaged tempting high-calorie food items conveniently and irresistibly in your face—they're winning the battle for your food habits.

Less-flashy-but-nutritious foods are being crowded out of your mind, your diet and your stores, in favor of highly manufactured concoctions engineered mainly to entertain your taste buds and sugarcoat your emotional cravings.

Your eating habits are very susceptible to the loud, colorful distractions of marketing. But like children, your habits are also yours to train and manage. If you let them run completely amuck, you mainly have yourself to blame for the ensuing disasters.

## WE, THE PEOPLE, HAVE A BIG FAT PROBLEM.

Obesity is growing at an alarming rate in adults and children. The percentage of young people who are overweight has more than tripled since 1980. Besides misery, in 2000 obesity resulted in $61 billion in direct medical costs and $56 billion in indirect costs, according to the U.S. Centers for Disease Control and Prevention.

We're a nation that believes in a free economy. We can't have a Boston Tea Party and dump all the baked goods containing partially hydrogenated fats into the harbor (along with the marketers who ply us with fattening foods.) "Let the buyer beware" still applies, and much depends on taking personal responsibility.

So what are you to do—especially if you've spent a fortune "trying everything?" Spare your pocketbook and save yourself much misery, because the answer is so, so simple.

## THE MAJORITY OF PEOPLE IN THE NATIONAL WEIGHT CONTROL REGISTRY HAD ONE WEIGHT CONTROL SUCCESS STRATEGY IN COMMON: THE HABIT OF KEEPING A FOOD DIARY.

Since 1994, these 5,000 volunteer enrollees from all walks of life, using all sorts of strategies, and faced with the same food temptations and distractions as the rest of us, have lost an average of 60 pounds and maintained the loss for 5 years on average. 89% used a combination of both physical activity and diet to keep their weight down. Did we mention that in this, the largest group of successful weight loss maintainers that has ever been studied, the majority cited keeping a food diary as the one success strategy they had in common?

1,685 OVERWEIGHT PEOPLE WHO THOUGHT THEY COULDN'T LOSE WEIGHT DID—AND THOSE WHO KEPT A DAILY FOOD DIARY LOST TWICE AS MUCH WEIGHT.

A Kaiser Permanente Center for Health Research study funded by the National Institutes of Health and reported in the August 2008 issue of the American Journal of Preventive Medicine was one of the largest and longest running weight loss maintenance trials ever conducted. It was also one of the few to recruit a large percentage of African Americans (44 percent.) This is important because African Americans have a higher risk of conditions, including diabetes and heart disease that are aggravated by being overweight.

Participants were asked to eat more fruits and vegetables and low-fat dairy, exercise more regularly, and turn in a food diary at weekly support group meetings. More than two thirds of the participants lost at least nine pounds, enough to reduce their health risks. The average weight loss after six months was approximately 13 pounds. Those who journaled daily lost twice as much weight as those who journaled once a week or less.

TWO PEOPLE ARE ON A MISSION TO MAKE IT FUN TO GET INTO THE DAILY HABIT OF KEEPING A FOOD DIARY.

Did we use the word "fun" in the same sentence as "food diary?" Yes we did. Because we (the mom/daughter team that created the color-coded journaling system behind this food diary and the successful Streaming Colors™ Fitness Journal) think it's a terrible shame that people lose so much time and money on methods that don't help them sustainably lose weight—while ignoring something as inexpensive and effective (hello—LOSE TWICE THE WEIGHT!) as the humble food diary.

We suspect it's because they think it's going to be a lot of writing drudgery, or that they're going to have to be perfect about recording every little detail of what they eat (and who's got time for that?) or that they'll start it, and then get distracted or lose interest.

That's why we use color-coding to make it fun, easy and motivating for you to get in the habit of communing with your food diary every day. We want to help you stay in what we call Lean Mode as consistently as possible.

For while detail has its place, consistency is king. The Kaiser Permanente study found that even if participants just jotted down a quick note or email on what they ate, the people who kept track most often lost the most weight. The ones who jotted something down every day lost nearly twice as much as those who didn't keep track.

The Lean Mode, Color Code system makes it even easier to stay in a journaling frame of mind. On your busy days, just highlight your eating and exercise high points. Journal in more detail when you have time.

And besides—what would you rather do? Pick up a pen and some highlighters and record what you've done for the day, or haul yourself onto the treadmill and sweat your way through an extra workout to make up for overeating?

## PEOPLE IN LEAN MODE AREN'T PERFECT, BUT THEY ARE IN THE HABIT OF PAYING ATTENTION TO THEIR FITNESS HABITS.

What is Lean Mode? Maybe it's easier to describe what it's not. Chances are you've been there.

Lean Mode is NOT willy-nilly throw-caution-to-the-wind mindless eating and deluding yourself that the calories aren't piling up and it just doesn't matter.

Lean Mode is NOT leaving your good fitness intentions to chance, or your carbs count to memory, or the actual amount of fat in those low-fat cookies to the impression you got from a quick glance at the label.

Lean Mode is NOT kidding yourself that someone else can fix your poor eating and exercise habits for you, or exert more effective control over you (long-term) than you can yourself.

Lean Mode is NOT eating like everyone else just because, well, that's how everyone else eats.

Call it self-reporting, honesty with oneself, self-awareness, self-responsibility, self-directed health improvement, self-control, self-motivation, or any other self word you can think of, Lean Mode draws out your eating and exercise habits very clearly for you. You can run, but you can't hide—from yourself in Lean Mode!

Lean Mode is that kick-start you might need to begin losing your first 100 pounds. Or it might be the fine tuning you need to lose that last 10 pounds. Here's what we know for sure: when we're in Lean Mode, tracking our eating and exercise, we're thinner. When we leave it to chance, we're not.

PEOPLE WHO GET INTO LEAN MODE PAY ATTENTION TO THEIR EATING AND EXERCISE CHOICES LONG ENOUGH TO ESTABLISH HEALTHY NEW HABITS THEY WON'T HAVE TO THINK ABOUT ALL THE TIME.

The longer you stay in Lean Mode, the longer you pay attention to small actions and repeat them often enough to make them habits you can live with…a comfortable, natural, sustainable part of your new lifestyle.

Lean Mode is your ticket off the dieting roller coaster. Even if you slide back a little, you still retain many of your improved habits. And you know how to get back on track with color.

Over the long run, Lean Mode is the easy way to do your small part to help ease the obesity crisis. It won't take us back to the 1950's, but it may help the next few decades look (and feel) better.

## CHIC PEOPLE KNOW THAT DESPERATION IS NEVER ATTRACTIVE.

And there's no spot anywhere in the Lean Mode Food Diary for coloring in such desperate measures as popping weird pills to lose weight, following extreme eating rituals, starving oneself to a too-low BMI, exercising oneself ragged, or doing other desperate things that don't come naturally to the rest of the human race.

"Healthy" is the new chic. Money can't buy it. But you can cultivate it, in a colorful, fun, sustainable way with the Lean Mode Food Diary—and of course, with a commitment to put your precious health first in your life and in your food journaling.

ONLY ONE PERSON HAS THE ULTIMATE POWER TO GET INSIDE YOUR HEAD AND CHANGE YOUR EATING AND EXERCISE HABITS.

It's not your trainer, your family, your best friend, or your partner. It's you (of course!) You just need the right tool, and you're already holding it in your hands.

With the Lean Mode Food Diary you use color to bring your eating choices out into the open where you can see and understand them.

This in turn helps you look inward, to your own behaviors, and in doing so take back some of your control from the marketing titans who are constantly yammering away and hammering away at your mind space.

You gain more control over the vital decisions on what you will ingest to nurture your body and determine your future health.

One of our Streaming Colors Fitness Journal users, Jan H. from Chicago, said it quite well:

*"When you are overweight, you feel out of control and ashamed. I started my first journal with a lot of goals but was only able to commit to doing one. I gave up drinking soda. I went for three months with only one color on my journal. When I reflected on what I had accomplished for three months straight, I realized that I had taken control. It empowered me to try another goal and then another. I am 60 pounds lighter now thanks to your journal. Thank you."*

On your own, you begin to take back control. You don't do it by spending money on over-hyped diet products, but by standing your ground and making better decisions each day so that you can keep coloring them in. You truly see that you can't just spend your way out of a weight problem.

With Lean Mode, the only willpower you really need is the willpower to report to yourself honestly every day. And if that seems daunting, well, we agree. Being honest with ourselves might be the biggest hurdle most of us face. The Lean Mode Food Diary

encourages you to jump that hurdle in living color. And it gives you ways to track and celebrate your consecutive journaling days, to help motivate you toward consistency.

Color your Lean Mode Food Diary every day to shape the you that you have always wanted to see!

## POWERFUL PEOPLE EXERCISE CONTROL THROUGH THEIR OWN CIRCLES—AND SO WILL YOU WITH THIS FOOD JOURNAL.

Power circles at the highest levels of government decide mega policies that affect everything from the availability, price and make-up of the food you eat to the allowable pollutants in the very air you breathe as you exercise.

People working within the power circles at state and city levels have been successful in ensuring, for example, that the number of calories in menu items will be clearly displayed to you, or that you have sidewalks and trails on which to walk and bike.

Your friends and family create a circle of influence over your eating and exercise habits, as shown in recent studies at Dartmouth College and the University of Warwick, UK. If your friends are heavy, there's a better chance you will be, too—and vice versa.

But true power begins at a personal level and circles outward from there. That's why we call the circles you color in every day in this diary to show you met your daily goals, your PowerCircles™.

Even if you slack off occasionally on recording your details (as we all do) your PowerCircles will help you stay in Lean Mode. Coloring them in will remind, reward, reinforce and motivate you in continuing to take healthy actions each day. And those healthy actions will accumulate to become the habits that empower your new lifestyle.

Your personal empowerment will eventually circle back to influence your friends, family and co-workers in their diet and exercise habits.

The healthier purchase decisions you make as a food consumer will dictate to even the most powerful food marketers the products they can best sell.

A strong, healthy, empowered citizenry will have a ripple effect within the policy-making circles at all government levels.

**So grab your highlighters and get ready to fill your PowerCircles and your FoodDots and all your other Lean Mode bubbles with color!**

CHANGE YOUR HABITS, CHANGE YOUR LIFE.

"Each of us must be the change we want to see in the world."

*Mahatma Gandhi*
*(1869 - 1948)*

> "A goal
> without a plan
> is just a wish."
>
> *Antoine de Saint-Exupery*
> *(1900 - 1944)*

# III.   Before You Begin,
# Set Up Your Stats & Quick Look-Up Pages

Color-coding makes the Lean Mode Food Diary quick and easy to use.

But in declaring war on their fat cells, some people like to track every single calorie, carb or fat gram. To save time and space making those entries on your Daily pages, you can calculate ahead of time the nutritional data of your favorite foods and recipes and record it on the Quick Look-Up pages that follow. People usually eat the same 30 to 40 foods over and over again, so it's worth your time to set up those pages. Then, try to improve your "short list" of foods by adding items from the Healthy Super-Foods Quick Look-Up Chart we've provided.

In Lean Mode, you're accountable to yourself. So rate your current habits, at right, and then again after 28 weeks.

How would you rate your eating habits in terms of controlling portion size and the overall amount of food you eat each day?

I'm doing everything wrong   ① ② ③ ④ ⑤ ⑥ ⑦ ⑧   I'm doing everything positive I can

Rate your eating habits in terms of the nutritional value and soundness of the foods you eat.

① ② ③ ④ ⑤ ⑥ ⑦ ⑧

How many hours of low intensity exercise do you get, on average, each week?

① ② ③ ④ ⑤ ⑥ ⑦ ⑧

How many hours of moderate (enough to break a sweat) to high-intensity exercise do you get, on average, each week?

① ② ③ ④ ⑤ ⑥ ⑦ ⑧

How many eight-ounce glasses of water do you drink each day?

① ② ③ ④ ⑤ ⑥ ⑦ ⑧

# Enter Your Starting **Stats**

DATE _____ / _____ / _____

Before starting this Lean Mode Food Diary, enter your important health and fitness stats.

Use the + or - column to show changes realized from your previous Lean Mode Food Diary, if you wish.

| | **+** | **-** | | | **+** | **-** |
|---|---|---|---|---|---|---|
| WEIGHT | | | HEART RATE | | | |
| HEIGHT | | | BLOOD PRESSURE | | | |
| BMI | | | TOTAL CHOLESTEROL | | | |
| % BODY FAT | | | HDL | | | |
| WAISTLINE | | | LDL | | | |
| | | | | | | |
| | | | | | | |
| | | | | | | |

# Half Year **Stats**

DATE _____ / _____ / _____

Come back to this chart at the end of your journaling period and enter your new stats for comparison.

| | **+** | **-** | | | **+** | **-** |
|---|---|---|---|---|---|---|
| WEIGHT | | | HEART RATE | | | |
| HEIGHT | | | BLOOD PRESSURE | | | |
| BMI | | | TOTAL CHOLESTEROL | | | |
| % BODY FAT | | | HDL | | | |
| WAISTLINE | | | LDL | | | |
| | | | | | | |
| | | | | | | |
| | | | | | | |

# Set Up Your **Quick Look-Up Food Charts**
To save time in your daily journaling, build a list of foods you eat most often.

| FOOD ITEM | SERVING SIZE | CALORIES PER SERV | TOTAL FAT/ SAT FAT | CHOLEST MG | SODIUM MG | CARBS GRAMS | FIBER GRAMS | SUGARS GRAMS | PROTEIN GRAMS | |
|---|---|---|---|---|---|---|---|---|---|---|
| | | | | | | | | | | |
| | | | | | | | | | | |
| | | | | | | | | | | |
| | | | | | | | | | | |
| | | | | | | | | | | |
| | | | | | | | | | | |
| | | | | | | | | | | |
| | | | | | | | | | | |
| | | | | | | | | | | |
| | | | | | | | | | | |
| | | | | | | | | | | |
| | | | | | | | | | | |
| | | | | | | | | | | |
| | | | | | | | | | | |
| | | | | | | | | | | |
| | | | | | | | | | | |
| | | | | | | | | | | |
| | | | | | | | | | | |
| | | | | | | | | | | |
| | | | | | | | | | | |
| | | | | | | | | | | |
| | | | | | | | | | | |
| | | | | | | | | | | |
| | | | | | | | | | | |
| | | | | | | | | | | |
| | | | | | | | | | | |
| | | | | | | | | | | |
| | | | | | | | | | | |
| | | | | | | | | | | |

You can get much of this information from food labels, calorie count books, or online.

# Lean Mode
## A **ColorCode Mode**™ Food Diary

| FOOD ITEM | SERVING SIZE | CALORIES PER SERV | TOTAL FAT/ SAT FAT | CHOLEST MG | SODIUM MG | CARBS GRAMS | FIBER GRAMS | SUGARS GRAMS | PROTEIN GRAMS | |
|---|---|---|---|---|---|---|---|---|---|---|
| | | | | | | | | | | |
| | | | | | | | | | | |
| | | | | | | | | | | |
| | | | | | | | | | | |
| | | | | | | | | | | |
| | | | | | | | | | | |
| | | | | | | | | | | |
| | | | | | | | | | | |
| | | | | | | | | | | |
| | | | | | | | | | | |
| | | | | | | | | | | |
| | | | | | | | | | | |
| | | | | | | | | | | |
| | | | | | | | | | | |
| | | | | | | | | | | |
| | | | | | | | | | | |
| | | | | | | | | | | |
| | | | | | | | | | | |
| | | | | | | | | | | |
| | | | | | | | | | | |

Fast food restaurants can also supply this information online or on-site.

# Note Your **Favorite Recipes & Food Combos**
To save time and space on your Daily pages, calculate the nutritional data of your favorite recipes here.

| RECIPE/INGREDIENT | AMOUNT | CALORIES | TOTAL FAT/ SAT FAT | CHOLEST MG | SODIUM MG | CARBS GRAMS | FIBER GRAMS | SUGARS GRAMS | PROTEIN GRAMS | |
|---|---|---|---|---|---|---|---|---|---|---|
| | | | | | | | | | | |
| | | | | | | | | | | |
| | | | | | | | | | | |
| | | | | | | | | | | |
| | | | | | | | | | | |
| | | | | | | | | | | |
| | | | | | | | | | | |
| | | | | | | | | | | |
| | | | | | | | | | | |
| | | | | | | | | | | |
| | | | | | | | | | | |
| | | | | | | | | | | |
| | | | | | | | | | | |
| | | | | | | | | | | |
| | | | | | | | | | | |
| | | | | | | | | | | |
| | | | | | | | | | | |
| | | | | | | | | | | |
| | | | | | | | | | | |
| | | | | | | | | | | |
| | | | | | | | | | | |
| | | | | | | | | | | |
| | | | | | | | | | | |

You can get much of this information from food labels, calorie count books, recipe books, or online.

# Lean Mode
## A **ColorCode Mode**™ Food Diary

| RECIPE/INGREDIENT | AMOUNT | CALORIES | TOTAL FAT/ SAT FAT | CHOLEST MG | SODIUM MG | CARBS GRAMS | FIBER GRAMS | SUGARS GRAMS | PROTEIN GRAMS | |
|---|---|---|---|---|---|---|---|---|---|---|
| | | | | | | | | | | |
| | | | | | | | | | | |
| | | | | | | | | | | |
| | | | | | | | | | | |
| | | | | | | | | | | |
| | | | | | | | | | | |
| | | | | | | | | | | |
| | | | | | | | | | | |
| | | | | | | | | | | |
| | | | | | | | | | | |
| | | | | | | | | | | |
| | | | | | | | | | | |
| | | | | | | | | | | |
| | | | | | | | | | | |
| | | | | | | | | | | |
| | | | | | | | | | | |
| | | | | | | | | | | |
| | | | | | | | | | | |
| | | | | | | | | | | |
| | | | | | | | | | | |
| | | | | | | | | | | |
| | | | | | | | | | | |
| | | | | | | | | | | |
| | | | | | | | | | | |
| | | | | | | | | | | |
| | | | | | | | | | | |
| | | | | | | | | | | |

Be sure to check out the Healthy Super-Foods Quick Look-Up Chart on the next page and add some of those foods to your diet.

# Make It a Goal to Add Foods From This
## Healthy Super-Foods Quick Look-Up Chart
To save you time we've already looked up the data on these health-promoting foods.

| FOOD ITEM | SERVING SIZE | CALORIES PER SERV | TOTAL FAT/ SAT FAT | CHOLEST MG | SODIUM MG | CARBS GRAMS | FIBER GRAMS | SUGARS GRAMS | PROTEIN GRAMS | |
|---|---|---|---|---|---|---|---|---|---|---|
| Acai | pure frozen 100g | 80 | 6 | - | 10 | 7 | 1 | - | 2 | |
| Almonds | 1oz=23 pcs. | 163 | 14 | - | - | 6 | 3 | 1 | 6 | |
| Apple | 1 medium | 95 | - | - | 2 | 25 | 4 | 19 | - | |
| Avocado | 1 whole | 322 | 29 | - | 14 | 17 | 13 | 1 | 4 | |
| Banana | 1 med. 7-8" long | 105 | - | - | 1 | 27 | 3 | 14 | 1 | |
| Beans | red, kidney 1/2 c. | 112 | - | - | 2 | 20 | 5 | - | 7 | . |
| Blueberries | 1 c. raw | 84 | - | - | 1 | 21 | 4 | 15 | 1 | |
| Broccoli | 1 c. chopped | 31 | - | - | 30 | 6 | 2 | 2 | 3 | |
| Buckwheat/ kasha | 1 c. cooked | 155 | 1 | - | 7 | 34 | 5 | 2 | 6 | |
| Cabbage | 1 c. chopped | 22 | - | - | 16 | 5 | 2 | 3 | 1 | |
| Cottage cheese | 1 c. low-fat 1% | 163 | 2 | 9 | 918 | 6 | - | 6 | 28 | |
| Kefir | 1 c., 1% | 110 | 2 | 10 | 125 | 8 | - | 8 | 14 | |
| Oatmeal | 1/2 c. | 150 | 3 | - | - | 27 | 4 | 1 | 5 | |
| Olives | about 6 medium | 32 | 3 | - | 230 | 2 | 1 | - | - | |
| Pomegranates | 3-3/8" dia. | 105 | - | - | 5 | 26 | 1 | 26 | 1 | |
| Spinach | 1 c. | 7 | - | - | 24 | 1 | 1 | - | 1 | |
| Sweet potatoes | 1 c. cubed | 114 | - | - | 73 | 27 | 4 | 6 | 2 | |
| Tuna | fresh yellowfin 4 oz. | 122 | 1 | 51 | 42 | - | - | - | 27 | |
| Yogurt | plain, low-fat 8 oz. | 154 | 4 | 15 | 172 | 17 | - | 17 | 13 | |
| Walnuts | 1 oz./ 14 halves | 185 | 18 | - | 1 | 4 | 2 | 1 | 4 | |
| Wild Alaskan Salmon | 4 oz. | 190 | 10 | 70 | 53 | - | - | - | 24 | |

USDA National Nutrient Database for Standard Reference

# Start Building Your
## Activity/Workout Quick Look-Up Chart
Make notes on your favorite routes, routines, events, etc.

| | | | | |
|---|---|---|---|---|
| | | | | |
| | | | | |
| | | | | |
| | | | | |
| | | | | |
| | | | | |
| | | | | |
| | | | | |
| | | | | |
| | | | | |
| | | | | |
| | | | | |
| | | | | |
| | | | | |
| | | | | |
| | | | | |
| | | | | |
| | | | | |
| | | | | |
| | | | | |

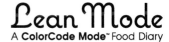

# Stepping Up To The New **Food Pyramid?**

Record your guidelines here.

The Lean Mode Food Diary works with just about any program. However, we don't endorse any particular program. Everyone has their own ideas, opinions, needs and style. That's why our system is versatile. And neutral. Like Switzerland.

The new Dietary Guidelines for Americans 2005 offer many food group based suggestions to help you toward a healthier lifestyle. If you'd like to track the new Food Pyramid with your Lean Mode Food Diary follow these steps:

**#1** Get your new customized USDA Food Pyramid Plan at MyPyramid.gov, or refer to the next page.

**#2** Decide on small, safe, realistic starting steps and goals. (Ask your doctor if you're not sure.)

**#3** Make necessary preparations for your new activities (e.g. buy the right exercise shoes, throw out the junk foods, buy healthy new foods, etc.)

**#4** Set up your Color Code and Goals in your Lean Mode Food Diary, based on recommendations from your chart at right.

**#5** Take action and color in your Lean Mode FoodDots and PowerCircles each day with the positive things you do.

**#6** Evaluate and reset your goals periodically so that you continue to improve and move in the direction of meeting more of your Food Pyramid Plan's guidelines. As certain foods or activities become habits you no longer need to think about or track, select new behaviors to improve.

**#7** If you fall away from your program, as many of us do at times, get back on track again as soon as possible. Look back on all that color and know that you have what it takes to improve.

---

## BUILD YOUR HEALTHY FOOD PYRAMID HABITS ONE COLORFUL DAY AT A TIME.

You can refer to the Quick Reference Charts on the next page, or get a customized plan at MyPyramid.gov*

My Pyramid Plan is based on a pattern of _____ calories per day

Fruits _____ cups

Vegetables _____ cups

Low-fat Milk _____ cups
(or equivalents)

Grains _____ ounces
(at least half should be whole grains)

Meats & Beans _____ ounces
(lean protein)

Healthy Oils _____ teaspoons

Limit extra fats & sugars to _____ calories

Total Fat _____ % of calories

Saturated Fat _____ % of calories

Cholesterol _____ mg

Sodium _____ mg

See MyPyramid.gov for full details of your recommended daily intake.

*My customized plan is based on info I entered on ___ / ___ / ___ at MyPyramid.gov

| Age | Gender | Height | Weight |

Physical Activity per Day:
○ Less than 30 minutes
○ 30-60 minutes
M○e than 60 minutes

# New **Food Pyramid** Quick Reference Chart

Follow these two steps to determine your daily food group amounts.

**MyPyramid.gov**
STEPS TO A HEALTHIER YOU

<table>
<tr><td style="width:28%; vertical-align:top;">

## STEP 1: LEARN HOW MANY CALORIES YOU SHOULD TAKE IN EACH DAY

See the USDA chart below for your estimated daily calorie needs. Or get complete details and your own customized plan at MyPyramid.gov.

Sedentary means a lifestyle that includes only the light physical activity associated with typical day-to-day life.

Active means a lifestyle that includes physical activity equivalent to walking more than 3 miles per day at 3 to 4 miles per hour, in addition to the light physical activity associated with typical day-to-day life.

</td></tr>
</table>

## STEP 2: STRIVE TO EAT THESE AMOUNTS DAILY FROM EACH FOOD GROUP

See the USDA chart below for your estimated daily calorie needs. Or get complete details and your own customized plan at MyPyramid.gov.

| CALORIE Level[1] | 1,000 | 1,200 | 1,400 | 1,600 | 1,800 | 2,000 |
|---|---|---|---|---|---|---|
| Fruits[2] | 1 cup | 1 cup | 1.5 cups | 1.5 cups | 1.5 cups | 2 cups |
| Vegetables[3] | 1 cup | 1.5 cups | 1.5 cups | 2 cups | 2.5 cups | 2.5 cups |
| Grains[4] | 3 oz–eq | 4 oz–eq | 5 oz–eq | 5 oz–eq | 6 oz–eq | 6 oz–eq |
| Meat/Beans[5] | 2 oz–eq | 3 oz–eq | 4 oz–eq | 5 oz–eq | 5 oz–eq | 5.5 oz–eq |
| Milk[6] | 2 cups | 2 cups | 2 cups | 3 cups | 3 cups | 3 cups |
| Oils[7] | 3 tsp | 4 tsp | 4 tsp | 5 tsp | 5 tsp | 6 tsp |
| Discretionary calorie allowance[8] | 165 | 171 | 171 | 132 | 195 | 267 |

| CALORIE Level[1] | 2,200 | 2,400 | 2,600 | 2,800 | 3,000 | 3,200 |
|---|---|---|---|---|---|---|
| Fruits[2] | 2 cups | 2 cups | 2 cups | 2.5 cups | 2.5 cups | 2.5 cups |
| Vegetables[3] | 3 cups | 3 cups | 3.5 cups | 3.5 cups | 4 cups | 4 cups |
| Grains[4] | 7 oz–eq | 8 oz–eq | 9 oz–eq | 10 oz–eq | 10 oz–eq | 10 oz–eq |
| Meat/Beans[5] | 6 oz–eq | 6.5 oz–eq | 6.5 oz–eq | 7 oz–eq | 7 oz–eq | 7 oz–eq |
| Milk[6] | 3 cups | 3 cups | 3 cups | 3 cups | 3 cups | 3 cups |
| Oils[7] | 6 tsp | 7 tsp | 8 tsp | 8 tsp | 10 tsp | 11 tsp |
| Discretionary calorie allowance[8] | 290 | 362 | 410 | 426 | 512 | 648 |

|  | **Sedentary** | **Active** |
|---|---|---|
| **Children** | | |
| 2–3 years | 1,000 | 1,400 |
| **Females** | | |
| 4–8 years | 1,200 | 1,800 |
| 9–13 | 1,600 | 2,200 |
| 14–18 | 1,800 | 2,400 |
| 19–30 | 2,000 | 2,400 |
| 31–50 | 1,800 | 2,200 |
| 51+ | 1,600 | 2,200 |
| **Males** | | |
| 4–8 years | 1,400 | 2,000 |
| 9–13 | 1,800 | 2,600 |
| 14–18 | 2,200 | 3,200 |
| 19–30 | 2,400 | 3,000 |
| 31–50 | 2,200 | 3,000 |
| 51+ | 2,000 | 2,800 |

1 **Calorie Levels** are set across a wide range to accommodate the needs of different individuals.

2 **Fruit Group** includes all fresh, frozen, canned, and dried fruits and fruit juices. In general, 1 cup of fruit or 100% fruit juice, or 1/2 cup of dried fruit can be considered as 1 cup from the fruit group.

3 **Vegetable Group** includes all fresh, frozen, canned, and dried vegetables and vegetable juices. In general, 1 cup of raw or cooked vegetables or vegetable juice, or 2 cups of raw leafy greens can be considered as 1 cup from the vegetable group.

4 **Grains Group** includes all foods made from wheat, rice, oats, cornmeal, barley, such as bread, pasta, oatmeal, breakfast cereals, tortillas, and grits. In general, 1 slice of bread, 1 cup of ready-to-eat cereal, or 1/2 cup of cooked rice, pasta, or cooked cereal can be considered as 1 ounce equivalent from the grains group. At least half of all grains consumed should be whole grains.

5 **Meat & Beans Group** in general, 1 ounce of lean meat, poultry, or fish, 1 egg, 1 Tbsp. peanut butter, 1/4 cup cooked dry beans, or 1/2 ounce of nuts or seeds can be considered as 1 ounce equivalent from the meat and beans group.

6 **Milk Group** includes all fluid milk products and foods made from milk that retain their calcium content, such as yogurt and cheese. Foods made from milk that have little to no calcium, such as cream cheese, cream, and butter, are not part of the group. Most milk group choices should be fat-free or low-fat. In general, 1 cup of milk or yogurt, 1 1/2 ounces of natural cheese, or 2 ounces of processed cheese can be considered as 1 cup from the milk group.

7 **Oils** include fats from many different plants and from fish that are liquid at room temperature, such as canola, corn, olive, soybean, and sunflower oil. Some foods are naturally high in oils, like nuts, olives, some fish, and avocados. Foods that are mainly oil include mayonnaise, certain salad dressings, and soft margarine.

8 **Discretionary Calorie Allowance** is the remaining amount of calories in a food intake pattern after accounting for the calories needed for all food groups—using forms of foods that are fat-free or low-fat and with no added sugars.

*Source: USDA web site MyPyramid.gov*
*07/25/05*

# CELEBRATE YOUR MILESTONES AND ACCOMPLISHMENTS WITH COLOR!

Color each circle or paste something in.

**Eat better.**
Did you break a
bad food habit, hit your
weight loss goal, fit into
your "skinny jeans,"
etc.?

**FILL THESE PAGES WITH COLOR ANY TIME OF THE YEAR.**

If it's important to you it's worth noting here!

**Exercise more.**
Did you meet your exercise goals, complete an event, set a new Personal Best, etc.?

"The journey
of a thousand
miles begins with
one step."

*Lao-Tse*
*(6th Century B.C.)*

# IV.   Getting Started & *Staying In* Lean Mode

Lean Mode puts a new spin on the food diary with daily FoodDots and PowerCircles, Weekly Tabs and 4Week Bubbles to which you add your own COLOR!

The Lean Mode Food Diary comes with just two rules, and leaves everything else up to you, like what to change and when to change, what to eat, goals, rewards, how much detail, and of course which colors to use!

## RULE #1: COLOR IN ONLY THE GOOD THINGS YOU DO.

You're trying to reward positive actions in order to repeat them often enough to crowd out your less desirable habits.

## RULE #2: COLOR IN SOMETHING EVERY DAY.

Consistency and small steps are the key to establishing healthy habits and losing more weight.

Throughout your Lean Mode Food Diary there are places to note and celebrate your days of continuous journaling.

Your diary is also undated, so that you can write in your own dates and get started at any time. Any day is a great day to switch your habits into Lean Mode.

The Lean Mode Food Diary is not your usual food diary because it offers you so much flexibility in what you track, in how much detail, and how you color or write it in. It works with any program.

Everyone does their diary differently, but here are a few filled-in sample pages to give you some ideas.

## WEEKLY COLOR CODE & GOALS PAGE

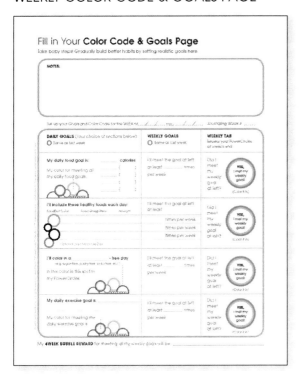

Your Lean Mode Food Diary starts every week with a Color Code & Goals Page that you can fill out—or ignore altogether and simply start recording things on your Food Diary Daily Pages. If you decide to set formal goals, your Color Code & Goals setting sections are self-explanatory and very flexible.

You can choose from a number of different types of goals. You can build flexibility into your weekly goal-setting by specifying how many days a week you'll meet your various daily goals. This is an important feature of the Lean Mode Food Diary. It allows you to set realistic goals and gradually improve. If you want to stick with your color code or goals a little longer, just select "same as last week."

But keep an eye on your goals. If you find your weight loss is slowing down, or you're not making as much progress, it might be time to make your goals a bit more challenging.

Make sure you've designated a reward for yourself (preferably not a high calorie treat. How about a massage, a new DVD, a movie with friends, or some new clothes?)

A popular feature of Lean Mode and all the Streaming Colors Fitness Journals is that they encourage you to color it in when you manage to skip a targeted food, e.g. a donut-free day, a candy-free day, or whatever food is your usual downfall. There's even a special, permanent spot for this in your PowerCircles. It's a practical way to gradually wean yourself off a food you're certain you can't live without.

## FOOD DIARY DAILY PAGE

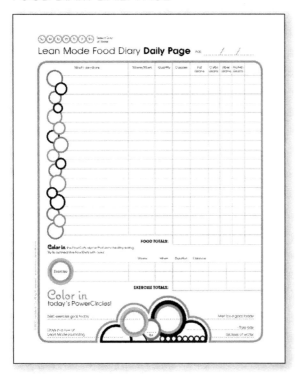

Every week there are seven Food Diary Daily Pages to fill in and total up. Starting out, you can keep it simple and just color in or write down when you do something positive to eat right or exercise. Even if you don't set goals, the act of recording what you're doing will give you insight, and also help you set some goals when you're ready.

If you want to use color to keep it simple, here's how extremely simple you could keep it. On your

first Daily page, just write in "Breakfast, Lunch, Dinner, or Snack" under the column heading "What I ate/drank."

If you felt it was overall a positive meal, color in the FoodDot on the same line. If not, leave it blank. If you don't see a lot of color, you'll know you have some tweaking to do. You can also color in the Exercise circle if you are active that day.

On the other end of the spectrum, you can write in everything you eat or drink in a day, including all pertinent nutrition facts. To save time, refer back to the Quick Look-Up Charts you filled in with the foods you frequently eat.

But don't stop there. Add some healthier foods to that list. To save you the trouble of looking them up, we've already included a Healthy Super-Foods Quick Look-Up Chart.

Here's a quick guide to filling out the columns on your Food Diary Daily Pages:

In the "WHAT I ATE OR DRANK" column you should enter:

- All food items you ate including condiments
- All beverages including alcohol
- Optionally: vitamins, supplements or meds you took

In the "WHERE/WHEN" column you could enter:

- Time of day
- Which meal — breakfast, lunch, dinner, snack. (If you are tracking by mealtimes, you may want to draw a squiggly line under the completed meal and subtotal your calories/carbs/etc.)
- General location such as home, work, car, restaurant, wedding, etc.
- Specific location such as at desk, at dining table, in bed, etc.
- Occasion such as out with friends, family dinner, (name of fast food restaurant) with the kids, etc.

This column can help you identify situations where you're likely to make poor food choices. Then you can develop strategies to avoid those situations and/ or alter the food choices you make in those situations.

In the "HOW MUCH" column enter:

- Quantity
- Number of servings, or
- Portion size

In the "CALORIES" column enter number of calories if you are tracking them.

In the "CARBS" column enter number of carbohydrate grams if you are tracking them.

Continue on across the columns to enter the categories you are tracking. There is one empty column to track a category of your own choosing. If you need to re-title some of the other columns just write over the existing column headings.

Regular exercise is vital to your overall health, as well as to weight loss and maintenance. There's a place on your Daily page to write in your activities and metrics.

Color in your Exercise circle to show you were active even if you didn't meet a daily exercise goal. If you wish to set a formal goal to color into your PowerCircles, objective measurements such as distance and duration are best. Consider using a pedometer to count your steps. If you want to compare your "calories in" to your "calories out," some treadmills and various wearable devices can give you an estimate of calories burned.

## ADD COLOR TO YOUR FoodDots

Each day color in the FoodDots next to the lines that you think show healthy eating. The more color you see there, the better you're doing.

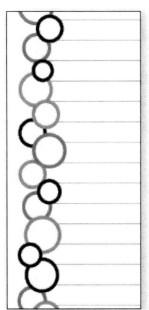

You could have special FoodDot colors for items such as:

- healthy food items (from our list or yours) that you are adding to your diet

- limiting yourself to healthy portions or quantities of a food

Now comes the fun part—connecting your FoodDots with COLOR!

Can you eat healthy all day long? If everything you ate was nutritionally sound, and you colored it in, you should have an unbroken chain of FoodDots for the day. That's quite an accomplishment, whether weight loss is your goal or not!

If you're seeing a lot of white in your FoodDots, hmmm. You might want to take a look at what you're eating and think about setting some small, reasonable goals for change.

Our FoodDots are forgiving! In your Color Code for the week, you can specify a color for foods that are neutral (not particularly healthy OR bad for you.)

You can also specify a color for a Lean Mode Lite day. That's a scheduled or unscheduled departure from your healthy eating.

Occasional exceptions are OK because they allow us to be human (holidays, being a gracious dinner guest, carbing up for an endurance event, etc.) without making us feel we've ruined our perfectly colored connect-the-FoodDots chain. They can also help us avoid slowing down our metabolism due to too few calories. So pick a color for your Lean Mode Lite days, but don't overdo them.

"Habit is habit, and not to be flung out of the window by any man, but coaxed downstairs a step at a time."

*Mark Twain*
*(1835 - 1910)*

## ADD COLOR TO YOUR PowerCircles

Every day, color your PowerCircles at the bottom of the daily page to reward your healthy actions and motivate yourself to keep it up! Make it as simple as you like, as long as it's meaningful to you!

Color in your PowerCircles to show you met your food or exercise goals, to track your weight, or to track how much water you drank. (We include a place to track water intake because water is so important to your overall health and vitality.) Or set a goal of your own. If you managed to avoid a specified food, write and color it in (e.g. a donut-free day, sugar-free day, etc.)

There's a circle to write in the number of consecutive days you've kept your journal or program going. Color it in to celebrate. If there's a break in your journaling, use a different color when you start over. (But do get started again!)

Color in your PowerCircles every day that you meet your specific goals, if you set them.

Congratulations! Every day that you do that is important in creating new habits! You will also refer back to these PowerCircles in tallying up your Weekly Tab, and then your 4Week Bubble and your Half Year Page. If you are motivated by long-term challenges, pay special attention to your PowerCircles.

If you're not seeing a lot of color in your PowerCircles, you may need to set more realistic goals. Or you may need to think about ways you can overcome some of the barriers that block your empowerment toward better habits. When you are truly in Lean Mode, you'll find you don't let much stand in the way of coloring in your PowerCircles.

All of the Lean Mode modules and pages are designed to be customized. There's just no one else on earth quite like you, so be your brilliant, creative self and make the circles your own, and/or use the guides we've suggested.

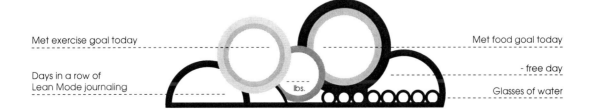

Met exercise goal today

Days in a row of Lean Mode journaling

lbs.

Met food goal today

- free day

Glasses of water

## REVIEW THE WEEK AND COLOR IN YOUR WEEKLY TAB

At the end of the week, look back over the days, review your PowerCircles and tally them up and see if you met your weekly goals. If so, color them in under your Weekly Tab! What an accomplishment!

Remember that in setting up your weekly goals, you didn't have to set a goal in every section, or be perfect every day. You were able to choose how many times a week you'd meet your various daily goals, a very flexible, forgiving and realistic way to set goals and rewards.

As your positive actions turn into habits, they'll come naturally to you and you can move on to track something else. (It's always something.) We know that if your goals get TOO easy to meet, you'll make them a little tougher for yourself next time. After all, it's your goal to keep improving.

| WEEKLY GOALS ◯ Same as last week | WEEKLY TAB Review your PowerCircles at week's end |
| --- | --- |
| I'll meet the goal at left at least _____ times per week | Did I meet my weekly goal at left? **YES,** I met my weekly goal! (Color it in) |
| I'll meet the goal at left at least _____ times per week _____ times per week _____ times per week | Did I meet my weekly goal at left? **YES,** I met my weekly goal! (Color it in) |
| I'll meet the goal at left at least _____ times per week | Did I meet my weekly goal at left? **YES,** I met my weekly goal! (Color it in) |
| I'll meet the goal at left at least _____ times per week | Did I meet my weekly goal at left? **YES,** I met my weekly goal! (Color it in) |

## COMPLETE YOUR 4WEEK BUBBLE RECAP

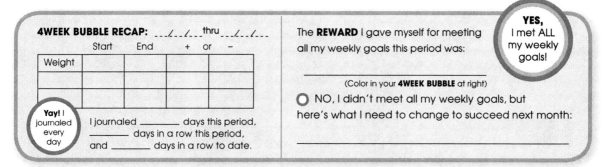

Now at the end of four weeks, you look back over your Weekly Tabs and see if you can color in your 4Week Bubble for having met all your weekly goals you chose to set.

Awesome, if you can! You are in maximum Lean Mode! Treat yourself to the reward you set up 4 weeks ago. Be sure to fill in your number of days of continuous journaling!

## YOUR HALF YEAR IN LEAN MODE

When you're out of Daily pages, it's time to fill in your Half Year Lean Mode pages. Color in all the 4Week Bubbles where you met your goals. Compare your changes from start to finish.

Congratulations on taking charge of your habits and improving them! We hope that Lean Mode has become your usual healthy mode, and that you are seeing the results you wanted to see!

Don't lose your momentum. Make sure you stay in Lean Mode by ordering another Lean Mode Food Diary right away!

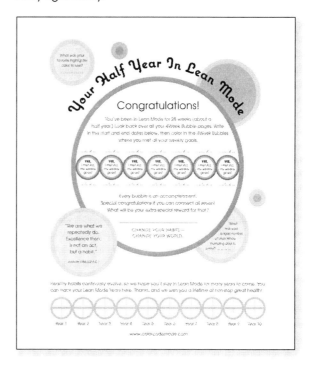

"Perhaps
the reward of
the spirit who tries,
is not the goal but
the exercise."

Edmund Vance Cooke
(1866-1932)

# V.   Lean Mode, Color Code Food Diary Pages

It's time to get into Lean Mode. Get out your highlighters and set your goals on the Color Code & Goals Page that follows.

Don't try to change all your habits at once, and be sure to consult with your doctor if you have any concerns about your diet, nutrition, or exercise choices.

Lean Mode doesn't recommend any particular diet or food plan, except to suggest that you try to get maximum nutritional value out of the calories you do take in. Avoid highly processed foods as they are full of hidden salt and sugar. (Don't keep them around your house to tempt you.) Get back to the basics and eat pure, wholesome foods.

Even if you don't need to lose weight, your body will always need exercise for optimal overall health and well being. Official recommendations vary, but in general

- for better health, accumulate 30 minutes of moderate-intensity physical activity five or more times a week

- for weight control, exercise 60 minutes at moderate intensity (or above) per day on average

If you're not yet ready to set goals, just start jotting down your eating and exercise choices on your Daily page (the page right after your Color Code & Goals Page) and color in the positive things you do. Seeing what you are currently doing will help you set goals in the future. You'll pick up the fine points of setting goals as you go along.

Be sure to keep track of your consecutive days of journaling! Consistency is one of your main goals.

Your completed Lean Mood Food Diary will be a colorful, completely unique picture of you... anything but your usual food diary!

# Fill in Your **Color Code & Goals Page**

Take baby steps! Gradually build better habits by setting realistic goals here.

**NOTES:**

Set up your Goals and Color Code for the WEEK of ___ / ___ / ___ thru ___ / ___ / ___   Journaling Week # _____

| **DAILY GOALS** (Your choice of sections below)  ○ Same as last week | **WEEKLY GOALS**  ○ Same as last week | **WEEKLY TAB**  Review your PowerCircles at week's end |
|---|---|---|
| **My daily food goal is:** _____ **calories**  My color for meeting all my daily food goals: ( )  ( )  ( )  ( ) | I'll meet the goal at left at least _____ times per week | Did I meet my weekly goal at left? **YES, I met my weekly goal!** (Color it in) |
| **I'll include these healthy foods each day:**  FoodDot Color    Food Group/Item    Amount  _Optional Lean Mode Lite Day_ | I'll meet the goal at left at least  _____ times per week  _____ times per week  _____ times per week | Did I meet my weekly goal at left? **YES, I met my weekly goal!** (Color it in) |
| **I'll color in a** _____ **- free day**  (e.g. sugar-free, pastry-free, soda-free, etc.)  in this color in this spot in my PowerCircles: | I'll meet the goal at left at least _____ times per week | Did I meet my weekly goal at left? **YES, I met my weekly goal!** (Color it in) |
| **My daily exercise goal is:** _____  My color for meeting my daily exercise goal is: | I'll meet the goal at left at least _____ times per week | Did I meet my weekly goal at left? **YES, I met my weekly goal!** (Color it in) |

My **4WEEK BUBBLE REWARD** for meeting all my weekly goals will be: _____

Su M Tu W Th F Sa  **Select Day of Week**

# Lean Mode Food Diary **Daily Page** FOR ___ / ___ / ___

| What I ate/drank | Where/When | Quantity | Calories | Fat Grams | Carbs Grams | Fiber Grams | Protein Grams |
|---|---|---|---|---|---|---|---|
| | | | | | | | |
| | | | | | | | |
| | | | | | | | |
| | | | | | | | |
| | | | | | | | |
| | | | | | | | |
| | | | | | | | |
| | | | | | | | |
| | | | | | | | |
| | | | | | | | |
| | | | | | | | |
| **FOOD TOTALS:** | | | | | | | |

**Color in** the FoodDots above that show healthy eating.
Try to connect-the-FoodDots with color.

| | Where | When | Duration | Distance | | |
|---|---|---|---|---|---|---|
| Exercise | | | | | | |
| **EXERCISE TOTALS:** | | | | | | |

## Color in today's PowerCircles!

Met exercise goal today ____

Days in a row of Lean Mode journaling ____

lbs.

Met food goal today ____

- free day ____

Glasses of water ____

# Lean Mode Food Diary **Daily Page** FOR _____ / _____ / _____

| What I ate/drank | Where/When | Quantity | Calories | Fat Grams | Carbs Grams | Fiber Grams | Protein Grams | |
|---|---|---|---|---|---|---|---|---|
| | | | | | | | | |
| | | | | | | | | |
| | | | | | | | | |
| | | | | | | | | |
| | | | | | | | | |
| | | | | | | | | |
| | | | | | | | | |
| | | | | | | | | |
| | | | | | | | | |
| | | | | | | | | |
| | | | | | | | | |

**FOOD TOTALS:**

**Color in** the FoodDots above that show healthy eating.
Try to connect-the-FoodDots with color.

| | Where | When | Duration | Distance |
|---|---|---|---|---|
| Exercise | | | | |

**EXERCISE TOTALS:**

## Color in
## today's PowerCircles!

Met exercise goal today _____

Days in a row of
Lean Mode journaling _____        lbs.

Met food goal today _____

- free day _____

Glasses of water _____

# Lean Mode Food Diary **Daily Page** FOR _____ / _____ / _____

| What I ate/drank | Where/When | Quantity | Calories | Fat Grams | Carbs Grams | Fiber Grams | Protein Grams | |
|---|---|---|---|---|---|---|---|---|
| | | | | | | | | |
| | | | | | | | | |
| | | | | | | | | |
| | | | | | | | | |
| | | | | | | | | |
| | | | | | | | | |
| | | | | | | | | |
| | | | | | | | | |
| | | | | | | | | |
| | | | | | | | | |
| | | | | | | | | |
| | | | | | | | | |
| | | | | | | | | |
| | | | | | | | | |
| | | | | | | | | |
| **FOOD TOTALS:** | | | | | | | | |

**Color in** the FoodDots above that show healthy eating. Try to connect-the-FoodDots with color.

| Exercise | Where | When | Duration | Distance | |
|---|---|---|---|---|---|
| | | | | | |
| **EXERCISE TOTALS:** | | | | | |

## Color in today's PowerCircles!

Met exercise goal today _____

Days in a row of Lean Mode journaling _____

_____ lbs.

Met food goal today _____

- free day _____

Glasses of water _____

# Lean Mode Food Diary **Daily Page** FOR _____ / _____ / _____

| What I ate/drank | Where/When | Quantity | Calories | Fat Grams | Carbs Grams | Fiber Grams | Protein Grams | |
|---|---|---|---|---|---|---|---|---|
| | | | | | | | | |
| | | | | | | | | |
| | | | | | | | | |
| | | | | | | | | |
| | | | | | | | | |
| | | | | | | | | |
| | | | | | | | | |
| | | | | | | | | |
| | | | | | | | | |
| | | | | | | | | |
| | | | | | | | | |
| | | | | | | | | |

**FOOD TOTALS:**

**Color in** the FoodDots above that show healthy eating.
Try to connect-the-FoodDots with color.

| | Where | When | Duration | Distance |
|---|---|---|---|---|
| Exercise | | | | |

**EXERCISE TOTALS:**

# Color in
## today's PowerCircles!

Met exercise goal today

Met food goal today

- free day

Days in a row of
Lean Mode journaling                    lbs.                    Glasses of water

Su  M  Tu  W  Th  F  Sa   Select Day
of Week

# Lean Mode Food Diary **Daily Page** FOR _____/_____/_____

| What I ate/drank | Where/When | Quantity | Calories | Fat Grams | Carbs Grams | Fiber Grams | Protein Grams |
|---|---|---|---|---|---|---|---|
| | | | | | | | |
| | | | | | | | |
| | | | | | | | |
| | | | | | | | |
| | | | | | | | |
| | | | | | | | |
| | | | | | | | |
| | | | | | | | |
| | | | | | | | |
| | | | | | | | |
| | | | | | | | |
| | | | | | | | |
| | | | | | | | |
| **FOOD TOTALS:** | | | | | | | |

**Color in** the FoodDots above that show healthy eating.
Try to connect-the-FoodDots with color.

| | Where | When | Duration | Distance |
|---|---|---|---|---|
| Exercise | | | | |
| **EXERCISE TOTALS:** | | | | |

## Color in today's PowerCircles!

Met exercise goal today _____

Days in a row of
Lean Mode journaling _____

_____ lbs.

Met food goal today _____

- free day _____

Glasses of water _____

Su  M  Tu  W  Th  F  Sa   Select Day
of Week

# Lean Mode Food Diary **Daily Page** FOR _____ / _____ / _____

| What I ate/drank | Where/When | Quantity | Calories | Fat Grams | Carbs Grams | Fiber Grams | Protein Grams | |
|---|---|---|---|---|---|---|---|---|
| | | | | | | | | |
| | | | | | | | | |
| | | | | | | | | |
| | | | | | | | | |
| | | | | | | | | |
| | | | | | | | | |
| | | | | | | | | |
| | | | | | | | | |
| | | | | | | | | |
| | | | | | | | | |
| | | | | | | | | |
| | | | | | | | | |
| | | | | | | | | |

**FOOD TOTALS:**

**Color in** the FoodDots above that show healthy eating.
Try to connect-the-FoodDots with color.

| | Where | When | Duration | Distance | |
|---|---|---|---|---|---|
| Exercise | | | | | |

**EXERCISE TOTALS:**

## Color in today's PowerCircles!

Met exercise goal today _____

Days in a row of
Lean Mode journaling _____

lbs.

Met food goal today _____

- free day _____

Glasses of water _____

Su M Tu W Th F Sa  Select Day of Week

# Lean Mode Food Diary **Daily Page** FOR _____ / _____ / _____

| What I ate/drank | Where/When | Quantity | Calories | Fat Grams | Carbs Grams | Fiber Grams | Protein Grams | |
|---|---|---|---|---|---|---|---|---|
| | | | | | | | | |
| | | | | | | | | |
| | | | | | | | | |
| | | | | | | | | |
| | | | | | | | | |
| | | | | | | | | |
| | | | | | | | | |
| | | | | | | | | |
| | | | | | | | | |
| | | | | | | | | |
| | | | | | | | | |
| | | | | | | | | |
| | | | | | | | | |
| | | | | | | | | |
| | | | | | | | | |
| | | | | | | | | |
| **FOOD TOTALS:** | | | | | | | | |

**Color in** the FoodDots above that show healthy eating.
Try to connect-the-FoodDots with color.

| | Where | When | Duration | Distance |
|---|---|---|---|---|
| Exercise | | | | |
| **EXERCISE TOTALS:** | | | |

# Color in
today's PowerCircles!

Met exercise goal today _____

Days in a row of
Lean Mode journaling _____

_____ lbs.

Met food goal today _____

- free day _____

Glasses of water _____

# Fill in Your **Color Code & Goals Page**

Take baby steps! Gradually build better habits by setting realistic goals here.

**NOTES:**

Set up your Goals and Color Code for the WEEK of ___/___/___ thru ___/___/___   Journaling Week # _____

| **DAILY GOALS** (Your choice of sections below) ○ Same as last week | **WEEKLY GOALS** ○ Same as last week | **WEEKLY TAB** Review your PowerCircles at week's end |
|---|---|---|
| **My daily food goal is:** _____ **calories** My color for meeting all my daily food goals: ( ) ( ) ( ) ( ) | I'll meet the goal at left at least _____ times per week | Did I meet my weekly goal at left? **YES, I met my weekly goal!** (Color it in) |
| **I'll include these healthy foods each day:** FoodDot Color    Food Group/Item    Amount *Optional Lean Mode Lite Day* | I'll meet the goal at left at least _____ times per week _____ times per week _____ times per week | Did I meet my weekly goal at left? **YES, I met my weekly goal!** (Color it in) |
| **I'll color in a** _____ **- free day** (e.g. sugar-free, pastry-free, soda-free, etc.) in this color in this spot in my PowerCircles: | I'll meet the goal at left at least _____ times per week | Did I meet my weekly goal at left? **YES, I met my weekly goal!** (Color it in) |
| **My daily exercise goal is:** _____ My color for meeting my daily exercise goal is: | I'll meet the goal at left at least _____ times per week | Did I meet my weekly goal at left? **YES, I met my weekly goal!** (Color it in) |

My **4WEEK BUBBLE REWARD** for meeting all my weekly goals will be: _____

# Lean Mode Food Diary **Daily Page** FOR _____ / _____ / _____

| What I ate/drank | Where/When | Quantity | Calories | Fat Grams | Carbs Grams | Fiber Grams | Protein Grams |
|---|---|---|---|---|---|---|---|
| | | | | | | | |
| | | | | | | | |
| | | | | | | | |
| | | | | | | | |
| | | | | | | | |
| | | | | | | | |
| | | | | | | | |
| | | | | | | | |
| | | | | | | | |
| | | | | | | | |
| | | | | | | | |
| | | | | | | | |
| | | | | | | | |
| | | | | | | | |
| | | | | | | | |
| **FOOD TOTALS:** | | | | | | | |

**Color in** the FoodDots above that show healthy eating.
Try to connect-the-FoodDots with color.

| | Where | When | Duration | Distance |
|---|---|---|---|---|
| Exercise | | | | |
| **EXERCISE TOTALS:** | | | | |

# Color in
## today's PowerCircles!

Met exercise goal today _____

Days in a row of
Lean Mode journaling _____

_____ lbs.

Met food goal today _____

- free day _____

Glasses of water _____

# Lean Mode Food Diary **Daily Page** FOR ____ / ____ / ____

| What I ate/drank | Where/When | Quantity | Calories | Fat Grams | Carbs Grams | Fiber Grams | Protein Grams | |
|---|---|---|---|---|---|---|---|---|
| | | | | | | | | |
| | | | | | | | | |
| | | | | | | | | |
| | | | | | | | | |
| | | | | | | | | |
| | | | | | | | | |
| | | | | | | | | |
| | | | | | | | | |
| | | | | | | | | |
| | | | | | | | | |
| | | | | | | | | |
| | | | | | | | | |
| **FOOD TOTALS:** | | | | | | | | |

**Color in** the FoodDots above that show healthy eating.
Try to connect-the-FoodDots with color.

| | Where | When | Duration | Distance | |
|---|---|---|---|---|---|
| Exercise | | | | | |
| | | | | | |
| **EXERCISE TOTALS:** | | | | | |

# Color in
## today's PowerCircles!

Met exercise goal today ____

Met food goal today ____

Days in a row of
Lean Mode journaling ____

____ lbs.

- free day ____

Glasses of water ____

# Lean Mode Food Diary **Daily Page** FOR _____ / _____ / _____

| | What I ate/drank | Where/When | Quantity | Calories | Fat Grams | Carbs Grams | Fiber Grams | Protein Grams | |
|---|---|---|---|---|---|---|---|---|---|
| | | | | | | | | | |
| | | | | | | | | | |
| | | | | | | | | | |
| | | | | | | | | | |
| | | | | | | | | | |
| | | | | | | | | | |
| | | | | | | | | | |
| | | | | | | | | | |
| | | | | | | | | | |
| | | | | | | | | | |
| | **FOOD TOTALS:** | | | | | | | | |

**Color in** the FoodDots above that show healthy eating.
Try to connect-the-FoodDots with color.

| | Where | When | Duration | Distance |
|---|---|---|---|---|
| Exercise | | | | |
| **EXERCISE TOTALS:** | | | | |

## Color in today's PowerCircles!

Met exercise goal today _____

Days in a row of Lean Mode journaling _____    _____ lbs.

Met food goal today _____

- free day _____

Glasses of water _____

Su M Tu W Th F Sa **Select Day of Week**

# Lean Mode Food Diary **Daily Page** FOR _____ / _____ / _____

| What I ate/drank | Where/When | Quantity | Calories | Fat Grams | Carbs Grams | Fiber Grams | Protein Grams | |
|---|---|---|---|---|---|---|---|---|
| | | | | | | | | |
| | | | | | | | | |
| | | | | | | | | |
| | | | | | | | | |
| | | | | | | | | |
| | | | | | | | | |
| | | | | | | | | |
| | | | | | | | | |
| | | | | | | | | |
| | | | | | | | | |
| | | | | | | | | |
| | | | | | | | | |
| | | | | | | | | |
| | | | | | | | | |
| **FOOD TOTALS:** | | | | | | | | |

**Color in** the FoodDots above that show healthy eating.
Try to connect-the-FoodDots with color.

| | Where | When | Duration | Distance | |
|---|---|---|---|---|---|
| Exercise | | | | | |
| | | | | | |
| **EXERCISE TOTALS:** | | | | | |

# Color in
## today's PowerCircles!

Met exercise goal today _____

Met food goal today _____

Days in a row of Lean Mode journaling _____

_____ - free day

lbs.

Glasses of water _____

# Lean Mode Food Diary **Daily Page** FOR _____ / _____ / _____

| What I ate/drank | Where/When | Quantity | Calories | Fat Grams | Carbs Grams | Fiber Grams | Protein Grams | |
|---|---|---|---|---|---|---|---|---|
| | | | | | | | | |
| | | | | | | | | |
| | | | | | | | | |
| | | | | | | | | |
| | | | | | | | | |
| | | | | | | | | |
| | | | | | | | | |
| | | | | | | | | |
| | | | | | | | | |
| | | | | | | | | |
| | | | | | | | | |
| **FOOD TOTALS:** | | | | | | | | |

**Color in** the FoodDots above that show healthy eating.
Try to connect-the-FoodDots with color.

| | Where | When | Duration | Distance |
|---|---|---|---|---|
| Exercise | | | | |
| **EXERCISE TOTALS:** | | | | |

# Color in
## today's PowerCircles!

Met exercise goal today _____

Days in a row of
Lean Mode journaling _____

_____ lbs.

Met food goal today _____

- free day _____

Glasses of water _____

# Lean Mode Food Diary **Daily Page** FOR _____ / _____ / _____

| What I ate/drank | Where/When | Quantity | Calories | Fat Grams | Carbs Grams | Fiber Grams | Protein Grams |
|---|---|---|---|---|---|---|---|
|  |  |  |  |  |  |  |  |
|  |  |  |  |  |  |  |  |
|  |  |  |  |  |  |  |  |
|  |  |  |  |  |  |  |  |
|  |  |  |  |  |  |  |  |
|  |  |  |  |  |  |  |  |
|  |  |  |  |  |  |  |  |
|  |  |  |  |  |  |  |  |
|  |  |  |  |  |  |  |  |
|  |  |  |  |  |  |  |  |
|  |  |  |  |  |  |  |  |
|  |  |  |  |  |  |  |  |
| **FOOD TOTALS:** |  |  |  |  |  |  |  |

**Color in** the FoodDots above that show healthy eating.
Try to connect-the-FoodDots with color.

| Exercise | Where | When | Duration | Distance |
|---|---|---|---|---|
|  |  |  |  |  |
| **EXERCISE TOTALS:** |  |  |  |  |

## Color in today's PowerCircles!

Met exercise goal today _____

Met food goal today _____

- free day _____

Days in a row of Lean Mode journaling _____

_____ lbs.

Glasses of water _____

# Lean Mode Food Diary **Daily Page** FOR ___ / ___ / ___

| | What I ate/drank | Where/When | Quantity | Calories | Fat Grams | Carbs Grams | Fiber Grams | Protein Grams |
|---|---|---|---|---|---|---|---|---|
| | | | | | | | | |
| | | | | | | | | |
| | | | | | | | | |
| | | | | | | | | |
| | | | | | | | | |
| | | | | | | | | |
| | | | | | | | | |
| | | | | | | | | |
| | | | | | | | | |
| | | | | | | | | |
| | | | | | | | | |
| | | | | | | | | |
| | | | | | | | | |
| | **FOOD TOTALS:** | | | | | | | |

**Color in** the FoodDots above that show healthy eating.
Try to connect-the-FoodDots with color.

| | Where | When | Duration | Distance |
|---|---|---|---|---|
| Exercise | | | | |
| **EXERCISE TOTALS:** | | | | |

## Color in
today's PowerCircles!

Met exercise goal today _____

Met food goal today _____

- free day

Days in a row of
Lean Mode journaling _____    lbs.

Glasses of water

# Fill in Your **Color Code & Goals Page**

Take baby steps! Gradually build better habits by setting realistic goals here.

**NOTES:**

Set up your Goals and Color Code for the WEEK of ____/____/____ thru ____/____/____ Journaling Week # _____

| DAILY GOALS (Your choice of sections below) ◯ Same as last week | WEEKLY GOALS ◯ Same as last week | WEEKLY TAB Review your PowerCircles at week's end |
|---|---|---|
| **My daily food goal is:** _____ **calories** <br> My color for meeting all ( ) <br> my daily food goals: ( ) <br> ( ) <br> ( ) | I'll meet the goal at left at least _____ times per week | Did I meet my weekly goal at left? **YES, I met my weekly goal!** (Color it in) |
| **I'll include these healthy foods each day:** <br> FoodDot Color    Food Group/Item    Amount <br> <br> <br> Optional Lean Mode Lite Day | I'll meet the goal at left at least <br> _____ times per week <br> _____ times per week <br> _____ times per week | Did I meet my weekly goal at left? **YES, I met my weekly goal!** (Color it in) |
| **I'll color in a** _____ **- free day** <br> (e.g. sugar-free, pastry-free, soda-free, etc.) <br> in this color in this spot in my PowerCircles: | I'll meet the goal at left at least _____ times per week | Did I meet my weekly goal at left? **YES, I met my weekly goal!** (Color it in) |
| **My daily exercise goal is:** _____ <br> My color for meeting my daily exercise goal is: | I'll meet the goal at left at least _____ times per week | Did I meet my weekly goal at left? **YES, I met my weekly goal!** (Color it in) |

My **4WEEK BUBBLE REWARD** for meeting all my weekly goals will be: _____

# Lean Mode Food Diary **Daily Page** FOR _____ / _____ / _____

| | What I ate/drank | Where/When | Quantity | Calories | Fat Grams | Carbs Grams | Fiber Grams | Protein Grams | |
|---|---|---|---|---|---|---|---|---|---|
| | | | | | | | | | |
| | | | | | | | | | |
| | | | | | | | | | |
| | | | | | | | | | |
| | | | | | | | | | |
| | | | | | | | | | |
| | | | | | | | | | |
| | | | | | | | | | |
| | | | | | | | | | |
| | | | | | | | | | |
| | | | | | | | | | |
| | | | | | | | | | |
| | | | | | | | | | |
| | | | | | | | | | |
| **FOOD TOTALS:** | | | | | | | | | |

**Color in** the FoodDots above that show healthy eating.
Try to connect-the-FoodDots with color.

| | | Where | When | Duration | Distance |
|---|---|---|---|---|---|
| Exercise | | | | | |
| | | | | | |
| **EXERCISE TOTALS:** | | | | | |

## Color in
### today's PowerCircles!

Met exercise goal today _____

Days in a row of
Lean Mode journaling _____

_____ lbs.

Met food goal today _____

- free day _____

Glasses of water _____

Su M Tu W Th F Sa  Select Day of Week

# Lean Mode Food Diary **Daily Page** FOR ___/___/___

| What I ate/drank | Where/When | Quantity | Calories | Fat Grams | Carbs Grams | Fiber Grams | Protein Grams | |
|---|---|---|---|---|---|---|---|---|
| | | | | | | | | |

**FOOD TOTALS:**

**Color in** the FoodDots above that show healthy eating.
Try to connect-the-FoodDots with color.

| | Where | When | Duration | Distance |
|---|---|---|---|---|
| Exercise | | | | |

**EXERCISE TOTALS:**

## Color in today's PowerCircles!

Met exercise goal today _____

Days in a row of Lean Mode journaling _____

lbs.

Met food goal today _____

- free day _____

Glasses of water _____

Su  M  Tu  W  Th  F  Sa   Select Day of Week

# Lean Mode Food Diary **Daily Page** FOR _____ / _____ / _____

| | What I ate/drank | Where/When | Quantity | Calories | Fat Grams | Carbs Grams | Fiber Grams | Protein Grams | |
|---|---|---|---|---|---|---|---|---|---|
| | | | | | | | | | |
| | | | | | | | | | |
| | | | | | | | | | |
| | | | | | | | | | |
| | | | | | | | | | |
| | | | | | | | | | |
| | | | | | | | | | |
| | | | | | | | | | |
| | | | | | | | | | |
| | | | | | | | | | |
| | | | | | | | | | |
| | | | | | | | | | |
| | | | | | | | | | |
| | | | | | | | | | |
| | | | | | | | | | |
| | **FOOD TOTALS:** | | | | | | | | |

**Color in** the FoodDots above that show healthy eating.
Try to connect-the-FoodDots with color.

| | Where | When | Duration | Distance | |
|---|---|---|---|---|---|
| Exercise | | | | | |
| **EXERCISE TOTALS:** | | | | | |

## Color in today's PowerCircles!

Met exercise goal today _____

Days in a row of Lean Mode journaling _____

_____ lbs.

Met food goal today _____

_____ - free day

Glasses of water _____

# Lean Mode Food Diary **Daily Page** FOR _____/_____/_____

| | What I ate/drank | Where/When | Quantity | Calories | Fat Grams | Carbs Grams | Fiber Grams | Protein Grams | |
|---|---|---|---|---|---|---|---|---|---|
| | | | | | | | | | |

**FOOD TOTALS:**

**Color in** the FoodDots above that show healthy eating.
Try to connect-the-FoodDots with color.

| | Where | When | Duration | Distance |
|---|---|---|---|---|
| Exercise | | | | |

**EXERCISE TOTALS:**

## Color in
## today's PowerCircles!

Met exercise goal today

Met food goal today

- free day

Days in a row of
Lean Mode journaling

lbs.

Glasses of water

Su  M  Tu  W  Th  F  Sa  Select Day of Week

# Lean Mode Food Diary **Daily Page** FOR _____ / _____ / _____

| What I ate/drank | Where/When | Quantity | Calories | Fat Grams | Carbs Grams | Fiber Grams | Protein Grams |
|---|---|---|---|---|---|---|---|
| | | | | | | | |
| | | | | | | | |
| | | | | | | | |
| | | | | | | | |
| | | | | | | | |
| | | | | | | | |
| | | | | | | | |
| | | | | | | | |
| | | | | | | | |
| | | | | | | | |
| | | | | | | | |
| | | | | | | | |
| | | | | | | | |
| **FOOD TOTALS:** | | | | | | | |

**Color in** the FoodDots above that show healthy eating.
Try to connect-the-FoodDots with color.

| | Where | When | Duration | Distance |
|---|---|---|---|---|
| Exercise | | | | |
| **EXERCISE TOTALS:** | | | | |

# Color in
## today's PowerCircles!

Met exercise goal today _____

Met food goal today _____

Days in a row of
Lean Mode journaling _____

_____ lbs.

- free day _____

Glasses of water _____

Su M Tu W Th F Sa  **Select Day of Week**

# Lean Mode Food Diary **Daily Page** FOR _____ / _____ / _____

| What I ate/drank | Where/When | Quantity | Calories | Fat Grams | Carbs Grams | Fiber Grams | Protein Grams | |
|---|---|---|---|---|---|---|---|---|
| | | | | | | | | |
| | | | | | | | | |
| | | | | | | | | |
| | | | | | | | | |
| | | | | | | | | |
| | | | | | | | | |
| | | | | | | | | |
| | | | | | | | | |
| | | | | | | | | |
| | | | | | | | | |
| | | | | | | | | |
| | | | | | | | | |
| **FOOD TOTALS:** | | | | | | | | |

**Color in** the FoodDots above that show healthy eating.
Try to connect-the-FoodDots with color.

| | Where | When | Duration | Distance |
|---|---|---|---|---|
| Exercise | | | | |
| **EXERCISE TOTALS:** | | | | |

# Color in
## today's PowerCircles!

Met exercise goal today _____

Met food goal today _____

_____ - free day

Days in a row of
Lean Mode journaling _____     ____ lbs.     Glasses of water _____

Su M Tu W Th F Sa    Select Day of Week

# Lean Mode Food Diary **Daily Page** FOR _____ / _____ / _____

| What I ate/drank | Where/When | Quantity | Calories | Fat Grams | Carbs Grams | Fiber Grams | Protein Grams |
|---|---|---|---|---|---|---|---|
| | | | | | | | |
| | | | | | | | |
| | | | | | | | |
| | | | | | | | |
| | | | | | | | |
| | | | | | | | |
| | | | | | | | |
| | | | | | | | |
| | | | | | | | |
| | | | | | | | |
| | | | | | | | |
| | | | | | | | |
| | | | | | | | |
| **FOOD TOTALS:** | | | | | | | |

**Color in** the FoodDots above that show healthy eating.
Try to connect-the-FoodDots with color.

| | Where | When | Duration | Distance | |
|---|---|---|---|---|---|
| Exercise | | | | | |
| **EXERCISE TOTALS:** | | | | | |

# Color in
## today's PowerCircles!

Met exercise goal today ..................... Met food goal today

..................... - free day

Days in a row of
Lean Mode journaling .....................    lbs.    Glasses of water

# Fill in Your **Color Code & Goals Page**

FILL THESE PAGES WITH COLOR   57

Take baby steps! Gradually build better habits by setting realistic goals here.

**NOTES:**

Set up your Goals and Color Code for the WEEK of ___ / ___ / ___ thru ___ / ___ / ___   Journaling Week # _____

| **DAILY GOALS** (Your choice of sections below) ⭕ Same as last week | **WEEKLY GOALS** ⭕ Same as last week | **WEEKLY TAB** Review your PowerCircles at week's end |
|---|---|---|
| **My daily food goal is:** _____ **calories** My color for meeting all my daily food goals: ( ) ( ) ( ) ( ) | I'll meet the goal at left at least _____ times per week | Did I meet my weekly goal at left? **YES,** I met my weekly goal! (Color it in) |
| **I'll include these healthy foods each day:** FoodDot Color   Food Group/Item   Amount _Optional Lean Mode Lite Day_ | I'll meet the goal at left at least _____ times per week _____ times per week _____ times per week | Did I meet my weekly goal at left? **YES,** I met my weekly goal! (Color it in) |
| **I'll color in a** _____ **- free day** (e.g. sugar-free, pastry-free, soda-free, etc.) in this color in this spot in my PowerCircles: | I'll meet the goal at left at least _____ times per week | Did I meet my weekly goal at left? **YES,** I met my weekly goal! (Color it in) |
| **My daily exercise goal is:** _____ My color for meeting my daily exercise goal is: | I'll meet the goal at left at least _____ times per week | Did I meet my weekly goal at left? **YES,** I met my weekly goal! (Color it in) |

My **4WEEK BUBBLE REWARD** for meeting all my weekly goals will be: _____

© 2009 Luna Media Co. All rights reserved. Lean Mode™ Forever Circles™ FoodDot™ are trademarks of Luna Media Co. www.colorcodemode.com

Su M Tu W Th F Sa  Select Day of Week

# Lean Mode Food Diary **Daily Page** FOR ____ / ____ / ____

| What I ate/drank | Where/When | Quantity | Calories | Fat Grams | Carbs Grams | Fiber Grams | Protein Grams |
|---|---|---|---|---|---|---|---|
| | | | | | | | |
| | | | | | | | |
| | | | | | | | |
| | | | | | | | |
| | | | | | | | |
| | | | | | | | |
| | | | | | | | |
| | | | | | | | |
| | | | | | | | |
| | | | | | | | |
| | | | | | | | |
| | | | | | | | |
| | | | | | | | |
| | | | | | | | |
| **FOOD TOTALS:** | | | | | | | |

**Color in** the FoodDots above that show healthy eating.
Try to connect-the-FoodDots with color.

| | Where | When | Duration | Distance |
|---|---|---|---|---|
| Exercise | | | | |
| **EXERCISE TOTALS:** | | | | |

# Color in
## today's PowerCircles!

Met exercise goal today _____

Met food goal today _____

- free day _____

Days in a row of Lean Mode journaling _____

lbs.

Glasses of water _____

Su  M  Tu  W  Th  F  Sa   Select Day
of Week

# Lean Mode Food Diary **Daily Page** FOR ___ / ___ / ___

| What I ate/drank | Where/When | Quantity | Calories | Fat Grams | Carbs Grams | Fiber Grams | Protein Grams | |
|---|---|---|---|---|---|---|---|---|
| | | | | | | | | |
| | | | | | | | | |
| | | | | | | | | |
| | | | | | | | | |
| | | | | | | | | |
| | | | | | | | | |
| | | | | | | | | |
| | | | | | | | | |
| | | | | | | | | |
| | | | | | | | | |
| | | | | | | | | |
| **FOOD TOTALS:** | | | | | | | | |

**Color in** the FoodDots above that show healthy eating.
Try to connect-the-FoodDots with color.

| | Where | When | Duration | Distance |
|---|---|---|---|---|
| Exercise | | | | |
| **EXERCISE TOTALS:** | | | | |

## Color in
today's PowerCircles!

Met exercise goal today _____

Days in a row of
Lean Mode journaling     lbs.

Met food goal today _____

- free day _____

Glasses of water

Su  M  Tu  W  Th  F  Sa  Select Day of Week

# Lean Mode Food Diary **Daily Page**  FOR _____ / _____ / _____

| What I ate/drank | Where/When | Quantity | Calories | Fat Grams | Carbs Grams | Fiber Grams | Protein Grams | |
|---|---|---|---|---|---|---|---|---|
|  |  |  |  |  |  |  |  |  |
|  |  |  |  |  |  |  |  |  |
|  |  |  |  |  |  |  |  |  |
|  |  |  |  |  |  |  |  |  |
|  |  |  |  |  |  |  |  |  |
|  |  |  |  |  |  |  |  |  |
|  |  |  |  |  |  |  |  |  |
|  |  |  |  |  |  |  |  |  |
|  |  |  |  |  |  |  |  |  |
| **FOOD TOTALS:** |  |  |  |  |  |  |  |  |

**Color in** the FoodDots above that show healthy eating.
Try to connect-the-FoodDots with color.

| Exercise | Where | When | Duration | Distance |
|---|---|---|---|---|
|  |  |  |  |  |
| **EXERCISE TOTALS:** |  |  |  |  |

# Color in
## today's PowerCircles!

Met exercise goal today _____

Days in a row of
Lean Mode journaling _____

_____ lbs.

Met food goal today _____

- free day _____

Glasses of water _____

# Lean Mode Food Diary **Daily Page** FOR _____ / ___ / _____

| | What I ate/drank | Where/When | Quantity | Calories | Fat Grams | Carbs Grams | Fiber Grams | Protein Grams | |
|---|---|---|---|---|---|---|---|---|---|
| | | | | | | | | | |
| | | | | | | | | | |
| | | | | | | | | | |
| | | | | | | | | | |
| | | | | | | | | | |
| | | | | | | | | | |
| | | | | | | | | | |
| | | | | | | | | | |
| | | | | | | | | | |
| | | | | | | | | | |
| | | | | | | | | | |
| | | | | | | | | | |
| | | | | | | | | | |

**FOOD TOTALS:**

**Color in** the FoodDots above that show healthy eating.
Try to connect-the-FoodDots with color.

| | Where | When | Duration | Distance | |
|---|---|---|---|---|---|
| Exercise | | | | | |

**EXERCISE TOTALS:**

## Color in
## today's PowerCircles!

Met exercise goal today _____

Met food goal today _____

Days in a row of
Lean Mode journaling _____        lbs.

_____ - free day

Glasses of water _____

Su M Tu W Th F Sa   Select Day of Week

# Lean Mode Food Diary **Daily Page** FOR ___ / ___ / ___

| What I ate/drank | Where/When | Quantity | Calories | Fat Grams | Carbs Grams | Fiber Grams | Protein Grams | |
|---|---|---|---|---|---|---|---|---|
| | | | | | | | | |
| | | | | | | | | |
| | | | | | | | | |
| | | | | | | | | |
| | | | | | | | | |
| | | | | | | | | |
| | | | | | | | | |
| | | | | | | | | |
| | | | | | | | | |
| | | | | | | | | |
| | | | | | | | | |
| | | | | | | | | |
| **FOOD TOTALS:** | | | | | | | | |

**Color in** the FoodDots above that show healthy eating.
Try to connect-the-FoodDots with color.

| | Where | When | Duration | Distance | |
|---|---|---|---|---|---|
| Exercise | | | | | |
| **EXERCISE TOTALS:** | | | | | |

## Color in today's PowerCircles!

Met exercise goal today _____

Met food goal today _____

Days in a row of Lean Mode journaling _____    lbs.

- free day

Glasses of water

Su M Tu W Th F Sa **Select Day of Week**

# Lean Mode Food Diary **Daily Page** FOR _____ / _____ / _____

| What I ate/drank | Where/When | Quantity | Calories | Fat Grams | Carbs Grams | Fiber Grams | Protein Grams | |
|---|---|---|---|---|---|---|---|---|
| | | | | | | | | |
| | | | | | | | | |
| | | | | | | | | |
| | | | | | | | | |
| | | | | | | | | |
| | | | | | | | | |
| | | | | | | | | |
| | | | | | | | | |
| | | | | | | | | |
| | | | | | | | | |
| | | | | | | | | |

**FOOD TOTALS:**

**Color in** the FoodDots above that show healthy eating.
Try to connect-the-FoodDots with color.

| | Where | When | Duration | Distance |
|---|---|---|---|---|
| Exercise | | | | |

**EXERCISE TOTALS:**

## Color in today's PowerCircles!

Met exercise goal today _____

Days in a row of Lean Mode journaling _____

_____ lbs.

Met food goal today _____

- free day _____

Glasses of water _____

Su M Tu W Th F Sa  Select Day of Week

# Lean Mode Food Diary **Daily Page** FOR _____ / _____ / _____

| What I ate/drank | Where/When | Quantity | Calories | Fat Grams | Carbs Grams | Fiber Grams | Protein Grams |
|---|---|---|---|---|---|---|---|
| | | | | | | | |
| | | | | | | | |
| | | | | | | | |
| | | | | | | | |
| | | | | | | | |
| | | | | | | | |
| | | | | | | | |
| | | | | | | | |
| | | | | | | | |
| | | | | | | | |
| | | | | | | | |
| | | | | | | | |
| | | | | | | | |
| **FOOD TOTALS:** | | | | | | | |

**Color in** the FoodDots above that show healthy eating.
Try to connect-the-FoodDots with color.

| | Where | When | Duration | Distance |
|---|---|---|---|---|
| Exercise | | | | |
| **EXERCISE TOTALS:** | | | | |

## Color in today's PowerCircles!

Met exercise goal today _____

Days in a row of Lean Mode journaling _____

lbs.

Met food goal today _____

- free day

Glasses of water

# Complete Your **4Week Bubble**

FILL THESE PAGES WITH COLOR   65

Look back over your Weekly Tabs for the past 4 weeks and tally the results.

**4WEEK BUBBLE RECAP:** ___/___/___ thru ___/___/___

Start        End        +   or   –

| Weight | | | |
|--------|--|--|--|
| | | | |
| | | | |
| | | | |

**Yay!** I journaled every day

I journaled _____ days this period,
_____ days in a row this period,
and _____ days in a row to date.

The **REWARD** I gave myself for meeting all my weekly goals this period was:

**YES,** I met ALL my weekly goals!

_____
(Color in your **4WEEK BUBBLE** at right)

○ NO, I didn't meet all my weekly goals, but here's what I need to change to succeed next month:

_____
_____

Set up your Goals and Color Code for the WEEK of___/___/___ thru ___/___/___   Journaling Week # _____

| **DAILY GOALS** (Your choice of sections below)<br>○ Same as last week | **WEEKLY GOALS**<br>○ Same as last week | **WEEKLY TAB**<br>Review your PowerCircles at week's end |
|---|---|---|
| **My daily food goal is:** _____ **calories**<br><br>My color for meeting all my daily food goals:<br>(   )<br>(   )<br>(   )<br>(   ) | I'll meet the goal at left at least _____ times per week | Did I meet my weekly goal at left?  **YES,** I met my weekly goal! (Color it in) |
| **I'll include these healthy foods each day:**<br>FoodDot Color        Food Group/Item        Amount<br><br>Optional Lean Mode Life Day | I'll meet the goal at left at least<br><br>_____ times per week<br>_____ times per week<br>_____ times per week | Did I meet my weekly goal at left?  **YES,** I met my weekly goal! (Color it in) |
| **I'll color in a** _____ **- free day**<br>(e.g. sugar-free, pastry-free, soda-free, etc.)<br>in this color in this spot in my PowerCircles: | I'll meet the goal at left at least _____ times per week | Did I meet my weekly goal at left?  **YES,** I met my weekly goal! (Color it in) |
| **My daily exercise goal is:** _____<br><br>My color for meeting my daily exercise goal is: | I'll meet the goal at left at least _____ times per week | Did I meet my weekly goal at left?  **YES,** I met my weekly goal! (Color it in) |

My **4WEEK BUBBLE REWARD** for meeting all my weekly goals will be: _____

© 2008 Luna Media Co. All rights reserved. Lean Mode™ PowerCircles™ FoodDots™ are trademarks of Luna Media Co.  www.colorcodenote.com

# Lean Mode Food Diary **Daily Page** FOR _____ / _____ / _____

| | What I ate/drank | Where/When | Quantity | Calories | Fat Grams | Carbs Grams | Fiber Grams | Protein Grams |
|---|---|---|---|---|---|---|---|---|
| | | | | | | | | |
| | | | | | | | | |
| | | | | | | | | |
| | | | | | | | | |
| | | | | | | | | |
| | | | | | | | | |
| | | | | | | | | |
| | | | | | | | | |
| | | | | | | | | |
| | | | | | | | | |
| | | | | | | | | |
| | | | | | | | | |
| | | | | | | | | |
| | | | | | | | | |
| | **FOOD TOTALS:** | | | | | | | |

**Color in** the FoodDots above that show healthy eating.
Try to connect-the-FoodDots with color.

| | Where | When | Duration | Distance | |
|---|---|---|---|---|---|
| Exercise | | | | | |
| | **EXERCISE TOTALS:** | | | | |

## Color in today's PowerCircles!

Met exercise goal today _____

Days in a row of
Lean Mode journaling _____

lbs.

Met food goal today _____

- free day _____

Glasses of water _____

Su M Tu W Th F Sa   Select Day
of Week

# Lean Mode Food Diary **Daily Page** FOR ___/___/___

| What I ate/drank | Where/When | Quantity | Calories | Fat Grams | Carbs Grams | Fiber Grams | Protein Grams | |
|---|---|---|---|---|---|---|---|---|
| | | | | | | | | |
| | | | | | | | | |
| | | | | | | | | |
| | | | | | | | | |
| | | | | | | | | |
| | | | | | | | | |
| | | | | | | | | |
| | | | | | | | | |
| | | | | | | | | |
| **FOOD TOTALS:** | | | | | | | | |

**Color in** the FoodDots above that show healthy eating.
Try to connect-the-FoodDots with color.

| | Where | When | Duration | Distance |
|---|---|---|---|---|
| Exercise | | | | |
| **EXERCISE TOTALS:** | | | | |

# Color in
## today's PowerCircles!

Met exercise goal today

Met food goal today

- free day

Days in a row of
Lean Mode journaling

lbs.

Glasses of water

Su  M  Tu  W  Th  F  Sa    Select Day of Week

# Lean Mode Food Diary **Daily Page**  FOR ___ / ___ / ___

| What I ate/drank | Where/When | Quantity | Calories | Fat Grams | Carbs Grams | Fiber Grams | Protein Grams | |
|---|---|---|---|---|---|---|---|---|
| | | | | | | | | |
| | | | | | | | | |
| | | | | | | | | |
| | | | | | | | | |
| | | | | | | | | |
| | | | | | | | | |
| | | | | | | | | |
| | | | | | | | | |
| | | | | | | | | |
| | | | | | | | | |
| | | | | | | | | |
| **FOOD TOTALS:** | | | | | | | | |

**Color in** the FoodDots above that show healthy eating.
Try to connect-the-FoodDots with color.

| | Where | When | Duration | Distance | |
|---|---|---|---|---|---|
| Exercise | | | | | |
| **EXERCISE TOTALS:** | | | | | |

## Color in today's PowerCircles!

Met exercise goal today ___

Met food goal today ___

- free day

Days in a row of Lean Mode journaling ___

lbs.

Glasses of water ___

# Lean Mode Food Diary **Daily Page** FOR ___ / ___ / ___

| What I ate/drank | Where/When | Quantity | Calories | Fat Grams | Carbs Grams | Fiber Grams | Protein Grams |
|---|---|---|---|---|---|---|---|
| | | | | | | | |
| | | | | | | | |
| | | | | | | | |
| | | | | | | | |
| | | | | | | | |
| | | | | | | | |
| | | | | | | | |
| | | | | | | | |
| | | | | | | | |
| | | | | | | | |
| | | | | | | | |
| | | | | | | | |
| | | | | | | | |
| | | | | | | | |
| | | | | | | | |
| | | | | | | | |
| **FOOD TOTALS:** | | | | | | | |

**Color in** the FoodDots above that show healthy eating.
Try to connect-the-FoodDots with color.

| | Where | When | Duration | Distance |
|---|---|---|---|---|
| Exercise | | | | |
| **EXERCISE TOTALS:** | | | | |

## Color in
## today's PowerCircles!

Met exercise goal today _____

Days in a row of
Lean Mode journaling _____

lbs.

Met food goal today _____

- free day _____

Glasses of water _____

# Lean Mode Food Diary **Daily Page** FOR _____ / _____ / _____

| | What I ate/drank | Where/When | Quantity | Calories | Fat Grams | Carbs Grams | Fiber Grams | Protein Grams | |
|---|---|---|---|---|---|---|---|---|---|
| | | | | | | | | | |
| | | | | | | | | | |
| | | | | | | | | | |
| | | | | | | | | | |
| | | | | | | | | | |
| | | | | | | | | | |
| | | | | | | | | | |
| | | | | | | | | | |
| | | | | | | | | | |
| | | | | | | | | | |
| | | | | | | | | | |
| | | | | | | | | | |
| | **FOOD TOTALS:** | | | | | | | | |

**Color in** the FoodDots above that show healthy eating.
Try to connect-the-FoodDots with color.

| | Where | When | Duration | Distance |
|---|---|---|---|---|
| Exercise | | | | |
| | | | | |
| **EXERCISE TOTALS:** | | | | |

# Color in
## today's PowerCircles!

Met exercise goal today _____

Days in a row of
Lean Mode journaling _____

_____ lbs.

Met food goal today _____

- free day _____

Glasses of water _____

Su  M  Tu  W  Th  F  Sa  Select Day
of Week

# Lean Mode Food Diary **Daily Page** FOR ___ / ___ / ___

| What I ate/drank | Where/When | Quantity | Calories | Fat Grams | Carbs Grams | Fiber Grams | Protein Grams |
|---|---|---|---|---|---|---|---|
| | | | | | | | |
| | | | | | | | |
| | | | | | | | |
| | | | | | | | |
| | | | | | | | |
| | | | | | | | |
| | | | | | | | |
| | | | | | | | |
| | | | | | | | |
| | | | | | | | |
| | | | | | | | |
| **FOOD TOTALS:** | | | | | | | |

**Color in** the FoodDots above that show healthy eating.
Try to connect-the-FoodDots with color.

| | Where | When | Duration | Distance | |
|---|---|---|---|---|---|
| Exercise | | | | | |
| **EXERCISE TOTALS:** | | | | | |

## Color in
today's PowerCircles!

Met exercise goal today _____

Days in a row of
Lean Mode journaling _____          _____ lbs.

Met food goal today _____

- free day _____

Glasses of water _____

# Lean Mode Food Diary **Daily Page** FOR _____ / _____ / _____

| | What I ate/drank | Where/When | Quantity | Calories | Fat Grams | Carbs Grams | Fiber Grams | Protein Grams | |
|---|---|---|---|---|---|---|---|---|---|
| | | | | | | | | | |
| | | | | | | | | | |
| | | | | | | | | | |
| | | | | | | | | | |
| | | | | | | | | | |
| | | | | | | | | | |
| | | | | | | | | | |
| | | | | | | | | | |
| | | | | | | | | | |
| | | | | | | | | | |
| | | | | | | | | | |
| | | | | | | | | | |
| | | | | | | | | | |

**FOOD TOTALS:**

**Color in** the FoodDots above that show healthy eating.
Try to connect-the-FoodDots with color.

| | Where | When | Duration | Distance | |
|---|---|---|---|---|---|
| Exercise | | | | | |

**EXERCISE TOTALS:**

## Color in today's PowerCircles!

Met exercise goal today _____

Met food goal today _____

- free day

Days in a row of Lean Mode journaling _____

lbs.

Glasses of water

# Fill in Your **Color Code & Goals Page**

Take baby steps! Gradually build better habits by setting realistic goals here.

**NOTES:**

Set up your Goals and Color Code for the WEEK of ____/____/____ thru ____/____/____   Journaling Week # _____

| **DAILY GOALS** (Your choice of sections below)<br>◯ Same as last week | **WEEKLY GOALS**<br>◯ Same as last week | **WEEKLY TAB**<br>Review your PowerCircles<br>at week's end |
|---|---|---|
| **My daily food goal is:** _____ **calories**<br><br>My color for meeting all<br>my daily food goals:<br>(    )<br>(    )<br>(    )<br>(    ) | I'll meet the goal at left<br>at least _____ times<br>per week | Did I<br>meet<br>my<br>weekly<br>goal<br>at left?   **YES,** I met my weekly goal!<br>(Color it in) |
| **I'll include these healthy foods each day:**<br>FoodDot Color    Food Group/Item    Amount<br><br>Optional Lean Mode Lite Day | I'll meet the goal at left<br>at least<br><br>_____ times per week<br>_____ times per week<br>_____ times per week | Did I<br>meet<br>my<br>weekly<br>goal<br>at left?   **YES,** I met my weekly goal!<br>(Color it in) |
| **I'll color in a** _____ **- free day**<br>(e.g. sugar-free, pastry-free, soda-free, etc.)<br>in this color in this spot in<br>my PowerCircles: | I'll meet the goal at left<br>at least _____ times<br>per week | Did I<br>meet<br>my<br>weekly<br>goal<br>at left?   **YES,** I met my weekly goal!<br>(Color it in) |
| **My daily exercise goal is:** _____<br><br>My color for meeting my<br>daily exercise goal is: | I'll meet the goal at left<br>at least _____ times<br>per week | Did I<br>meet<br>my<br>weekly<br>goal<br>at left?   **YES,** I met my weekly goal!<br>(Color it in) |

My **4WEEK BUBBLE REWARD** for meeting all my weekly goals will be: _____

# Lean Mode Food Diary **Daily Page** FOR ___ / ___ / ___

| | What I ate/drank | Where/When | Quantity | Calories | Fat Grams | Carbs Grams | Fiber Grams | Protein Grams | |
|---|---|---|---|---|---|---|---|---|---|
| | | | | | | | | | |
| | | | | | | | | | |
| | | | | | | | | | |
| | | | | | | | | | |
| | | | | | | | | | |
| | | | | | | | | | |
| | | | | | | | | | |
| | | | | | | | | | |
| | | | | | | | | | |
| | | | | | | | | | |
| | | | | | | | | | |
| | **FOOD TOTALS:** | | | | | | | | |

**Color in** the FoodDots above that show healthy eating.
Try to connect-the-FoodDots with color.

| | Where | When | Duration | Distance | | |
|---|---|---|---|---|---|---|
| Exercise | | | | | | |
| **EXERCISE TOTALS:** | | | | | | |

# Color in
## today's PowerCircles!

Met exercise goal today ___

Met food goal today ___

- free day ___

Days in a row of
Lean Mode journaling ___

lbs.

Glasses of water ___

Su  M  Tu  W  Th  F  Sa  Select Day
of Week

# Lean Mode Food Diary **Daily Page** FOR ___/___/___

| What I ate/drank | Where/When | Quantity | Calories | Fat Grams | Carbs Grams | Fiber Grams | Protein Grams | |
|---|---|---|---|---|---|---|---|---|
| | | | | | | | | |
| | | | | | | | | |
| | | | | | | | | |
| | | | | | | | | |
| | | | | | | | | |
| | | | | | | | | |
| | | | | | | | | |
| | | | | | | | | |
| | | | | | | | | |
| | | | | | | | | |
| | | | | | | | | |
| | | | | | | | | |
| | | | | | | | | |
| | | | | | | | | |
| **FOOD TOTALS:** | | | | | | | | |

**Color in** the FoodDots above that show healthy eating.
Try to connect-the-FoodDots with color.

| | Where | When | Duration | Distance | |
|---|---|---|---|---|---|
| Exercise | | | | | |
| **EXERCISE TOTALS:** | | | | | |

# Color in
## today's PowerCircles!

Met exercise goal today ___

Days in a row of
Lean Mode journaling ___

___ lbs.

Met food goal today ___

- free day ___

Glasses of water ___

Su  M  Tu  W  Th  F  Sa   Select Day of Week

# Lean Mode Food Diary **Daily Page** FOR _____ / _____ / _____

| What I ate/drank | Where/When | Quantity | Calories | Fat Grams | Carbs Grams | Fiber Grams | Protein Grams |
|---|---|---|---|---|---|---|---|
| | | | | | | | |
| | | | | | | | |
| | | | | | | | |
| | | | | | | | |
| | | | | | | | |
| | | | | | | | |
| | | | | | | | |
| | | | | | | | |
| | | | | | | | |
| | | | | | | | |
| | | | | | | | |
| | | | | | | | |
| | | | | | | | |
| **FOOD TOTALS:** | | | | | | | |

**Color in** the FoodDots above that show healthy eating.
Try to connect-the-FoodDots with color.

| | Where | When | Duration | Distance | | |
|---|---|---|---|---|---|---|
| Exercise | | | | | | |
| **EXERCISE TOTALS:** | | | | | | |

## Color in
### today's PowerCircles!

Met exercise goal today _____

Met food goal today _____

- free day

Days in a row of
Lean Mode journaling _____   lbs.   Glasses of water

Su M Tu W Th F Sa **Select Day of Week**

# Lean Mode Food Diary **Daily Page** FOR ___ / ___ / ___

| What I ate/drank | Where/When | Quantity | Calories | Fat Grams | Carbs Grams | Fiber Grams | Protein Grams | |
|---|---|---|---|---|---|---|---|---|
| | | | | | | | | |
| | | | | | | | | |
| | | | | | | | | |
| | | | | | | | | |
| | | | | | | | | |
| | | | | | | | | |
| | | | | | | | | |
| | | | | | | | | |
| | | | | | | | | |
| | | | | | | | | |
| | | | | | | | | |
| | | | | | | | | |
| | | | | | | | | |
| | | | | | | | | |
| **FOOD TOTALS:** | | | | | | | | |

**Color in** the FoodDots above that show healthy eating.
Try to connect-the-FoodDots with color.

| | Where | When | Duration | Distance | |
|---|---|---|---|---|---|
| Exercise | | | | | |
| **EXERCISE TOTALS:** | | | | | |

## Color in today's PowerCircles!

Met exercise goal today _____

Days in a row of Lean Mode journaling _____

_____ lbs.

Met food goal today _____

_____ - free day

Glasses of water _____

# Lean Mode Food Diary **Daily Page** FOR ____ / ____ / ____

| | What I ate/drank | Where/When | Quantity | Calories | Fat Grams | Carbs Grams | Fiber Grams | Protein Grams |
|---|---|---|---|---|---|---|---|---|
| | | | | | | | | |
| | | | | | | | | |
| | | | | | | | | |
| | | | | | | | | |
| | | | | | | | | |
| | | | | | | | | |
| | | | | | | | | |
| | | | | | | | | |
| | | | | | | | | |
| | | | | | | | | |
| | | | | | | | | |
| | | | | | | | | |
| | **FOOD TOTALS:** | | | | | | | |

**Color in** the FoodDots above that show healthy eating.
Try to connect-the-FoodDots with color.

| | Where | When | Duration | Distance |
|---|---|---|---|---|
| Exercise | | | | |
| **EXERCISE TOTALS:** | | | | |

# Color in
## today's PowerCircles!

Met exercise goal today _____

Met food goal today _____

- free day _____

Days in a row of
Lean Mode journaling _____

lbs.

Glasses of water _____

Su M Tu W Th F Sa  Select Day of Week

# Lean Mode Food Diary **Daily Page** FOR ___ / ___ / ___

| What I ate/drank | Where/When | Quantity | Calories | Fat Grams | Carbs Grams | Fiber Grams | Protein Grams | |
|---|---|---|---|---|---|---|---|---|
| | | | | | | | | |
| | | | | | | | | |
| | | | | | | | | |
| | | | | | | | | |
| | | | | | | | | |
| | | | | | | | | |
| | | | | | | | | |
| | | | | | | | | |
| | | | | | | | | |
| | | | | | | | | |
| | | | | | | | | |
| | | | | | | | | |
| | | | | | | | | |
| **FOOD TOTALS:** | | | | | | | | |

**Color in** the FoodDots above that show healthy eating.
Try to connect-the-FoodDots with color.

| | Where | When | Duration | Distance |
|---|---|---|---|---|
| Exercise | | | | |
| **EXERCISE TOTALS:** | | | | |

## Color in today's PowerCircles!

Met exercise goal today ___

Met food goal today ___

Days in a row of Lean Mode journaling ___

lbs.

- free day ___

Glasses of water ___

Su M Tu W Th F Sa    Select Day of Week

# Lean Mode Food Diary **Daily Page** FOR _____/_____/_____

| | What I ate/drank | Where/When | Quantity | Calories | Fat Grams | Carbs Grams | Fiber Grams | Protein Grams | |
|---|---|---|---|---|---|---|---|---|---|
| | | | | | | | | | |
| | | | | | | | | | |
| | | | | | | | | | |
| | | | | | | | | | |
| | | | | | | | | | |
| | | | | | | | | | |
| | | | | | | | | | |
| | | | | | | | | | |
| | | | | | | | | | |
| | | | | | | | | | |
| | | | | | | | | | |
| | | | | | | | | | |
| | **FOOD TOTALS:** | | | | | | | | |

**Color in** the FoodDots above that show healthy eating.
Try to connect-the-FoodDots with color.

| | Where | When | Duration | Distance |
|---|---|---|---|---|
| Exercise | | | | |
| **EXERCISE TOTALS:** | | | | |

# Color in
## today's PowerCircles!

Met exercise goal today _____

Days in a row of
Lean Mode journaling _____

lbs.

Met food goal today _____

- free day _____

Glasses of water _____

# Fill in Your **Color Code & Goals Page**

Take baby steps! Gradually build better habits by setting realistic goals here.

**NOTES:**

Set up your Goals and Color Code for the WEEK of____/____/____ thru ____/____/____ Journaling Week # _____

| **DAILY GOALS** (Your choice of sections below) ○ Same as last week | **WEEKLY GOALS** ○ Same as last week | **WEEKLY TAB** Review your PowerCircles at week's end |
|---|---|---|
| **My daily food goal is:** _____ **calories** My color for meeting all my daily food goals: ( ) ( ) ( ) ( ) | I'll meet the goal at left at least _____ times per week | Did I meet my weekly goal at left? **YES,** I met my weekly goal! (Color it in) |
| **I'll include these healthy foods each day:** FoodDot Color    Food Group/Item    Amount *Optional Lean Mode Lite Day* | I'll meet the goal at left at least _____ times per week _____ times per week _____ times per week | Did I meet my weekly goal at left? **YES,** I met my weekly goal! (Color it in) |
| **I'll color in a** _____ **- free day** (e.g. sugar-free, pastry-free, soda-free, etc.) in this color in this spot in my PowerCircles: | I'll meet the goal at left at least _____ times per week | Did I meet my weekly goal at left? **YES,** I met my weekly goal! (Color it in) |
| **My daily exercise goal is:** _____ My color for meeting my daily exercise goal is: | I'll meet the goal at left at least _____ times per week | Did I meet my weekly goal at left? **YES,** I met my weekly goal! (Color it in) |

My **4WEEK BUBBLE REWARD** for meeting all my weekly goals will be: _____

Su  M  Tu  W  Th  F  Sa   Select Day of Week

# Lean Mode Food Diary **Daily Page** FOR _____ / _____ / _____

| What I ate/drank | Where/When | Quantity | Calories | Fat Grams | Carbs Grams | Fiber Grams | Protein Grams | |
|---|---|---|---|---|---|---|---|---|
| | | | | | | | | |
| | | | | | | | | |
| | | | | | | | | |
| | | | | | | | | |
| | | | | | | | | |
| | | | | | | | | |
| | | | | | | | | |
| | | | | | | | | |
| | | | | | | | | |
| | | | | | | | | |
| | | | | | | | | |
| | | | | | | | | |
| | | | | | | | | |
| | | | | | | | | |
| | | | | | | | | |
| **FOOD TOTALS:** | | | | | | | | |

**Color in** the FoodDots above that show healthy eating.
Try to connect-the-FoodDots with color.

| | Where | When | Duration | Distance | |
|---|---|---|---|---|---|
| Exercise | | | | | |
| **EXERCISE TOTALS:** | | | | | |

## Color in today's PowerCircles!

Met exercise goal today _____

Met food goal today _____

_____ - free day

Days in a row of Lean Mode journaling _____

lbs.

Glasses of water _____

# Lean Mode Food Diary **Daily Page** FOR _____ / _____ / _____

| What I ate/drank | Where/When | Quantity | Calories | Fat Grams | Carbs Grams | Fiber Grams | Protein Grams | |
|---|---|---|---|---|---|---|---|---|
| | | | | | | | | |
| | | | | | | | | |
| | | | | | | | | |
| | | | | | | | | |
| | | | | | | | | |
| | | | | | | | | |
| | | | | | | | | |
| | | | | | | | | |
| | | | | | | | | |
| | | | | | | | | |
| | | | | | | | | |
| | | | | | | | | |
| | | | | | | | | |
| **FOOD TOTALS:** | | | | | | | | |

**Color in** the FoodDots above that show healthy eating.
Try to connect-the-FoodDots with color.

| | Where | When | Duration | Distance | |
|---|---|---|---|---|---|
| Exercise | | | | | |
| | | | | | |
| **EXERCISE TOTALS:** | | | | | |

## Color in today's PowerCircles!

Met exercise goal today _____

Days in a row of
Lean Mode journaling _____

_____ lbs.

Met food goal today _____

- free day _____

Glasses of water _____

Su M Tu W Th F Sa Select Day of Week

# Lean Mode Food Diary **Daily Page** FOR ___ / ___ / ___

| What I ate/drank | Where/When | Quantity | Calories | Fat Grams | Carbs Grams | Fiber Grams | Protein Grams |
|---|---|---|---|---|---|---|---|
| | | | | | | | |
| | | | | | | | |
| | | | | | | | |
| | | | | | | | |
| | | | | | | | |
| | | | | | | | |
| | | | | | | | |
| | | | | | | | |
| | | | | | | | |
| | | | | | | | |
| | | | | | | | |
| | | | | | | | |
| | | | | | | | |
| | | | | | | | |
| **FOOD TOTALS:** | | | | | | | |

**Color in** the FoodDots above that show healthy eating.
Try to connect-the-FoodDots with color.

| | Where | When | Duration | Distance |
|---|---|---|---|---|
| Exercise | | | | |
| **EXERCISE TOTALS:** | | | | |

# Color in
## today's PowerCircles!

Met exercise goal today ___

Met food goal today ___

- free day

Days in a row of
Lean Mode journaling ___     lbs.

Glasses of water ___

# Lean Mode Food Diary **Daily Page** FOR _____ / ____ / _____

| | What I ate/drank | Where/When | Quantity | Calories | Fat Grams | Carbs Grams | Fiber Grams | Protein Grams | |
|---|---|---|---|---|---|---|---|---|---|
| | | | | | | | | | |
| | | | | | | | | | |
| | | | | | | | | | |
| | | | | | | | | | |
| | | | | | | | | | |
| | | | | | | | | | |
| | | | | | | | | | |
| | | | | | | | | | |
| | | | | | | | | | |
| | | | | | | | | | |
| | | | | | | | | | |
| | | | | | | | | | |
| | | | | | | | | | |
| | **FOOD TOTALS:** | | | | | | | | |

**Color in** the FoodDots above that show healthy eating.
Try to connect-the-FoodDots with color.

| | Where | When | Duration | Distance |
|---|---|---|---|---|
| Exercise | | | | |
| **EXERCISE TOTALS:** | | | | |

# Color in
## today's PowerCircles!

Met exercise goal today _____

Days in a row of
Lean Mode journaling _____

_____ lbs.

Met food goal today _____

_____ - free day

Glasses of water _____

Su M Tu W Th F Sa  Select Day of Week

# Lean Mode Food Diary **Daily Page** FOR ___ / ___ / ___

| What I ate/drank | Where/When | Quantity | Calories | Fat Grams | Carbs Grams | Fiber Grams | Protein Grams | |
|---|---|---|---|---|---|---|---|---|
| | | | | | | | | |
| | | | | | | | | |
| | | | | | | | | |
| | | | | | | | | |
| | | | | | | | | |
| | | | | | | | | |
| | | | | | | | | |
| | | | | | | | | |
| | | | | | | | | |
| | | | | | | | | |
| | | | | | | | | |
| | | | | | | | | |
| | | | | | | | | |
| **FOOD TOTALS:** | | | | | | | | |

**Color in** the FoodDots above that show healthy eating.
Try to connect-the-FoodDots with color.

| | Where | When | Duration | Distance | |
|---|---|---|---|---|---|
| Exercise | | | | | |
| **EXERCISE TOTALS:** | | | | | |

## Color in today's PowerCircles!

Met exercise goal today _____

Met food goal today _____

- free day _____

Days in a row of Lean Mode journaling _____

lbs.

Glasses of water _____

( Su )( M )( Tu )( W )( Th )( F )( Sa )  Select Day
of Week

# Lean Mode Food Diary **Daily Page** FOR _____ / _____ / _____

| | What I ate/drank | Where/When | Quantity | Calories | Fat Grams | Carbs Grams | Fiber Grams | Protein Grams | |
|---|---|---|---|---|---|---|---|---|---|
| | | | | | | | | | |
| | | | | | | | | | |
| | | | | | | | | | |
| | | | | | | | | | |
| | | | | | | | | | |
| | | | | | | | | | |
| | | | | | | | | | |
| | | | | | | | | | |
| | | | | | | | | | |
| | | | | | | | | | |
| | | | | | | | | | |
| | | | | | | | | | |
| | | | | | | | | | |
| | | | | | | | | | |
| | **FOOD TOTALS:** | | | | | | | | |

**Color in** the FoodDots above that show healthy eating.
Try to connect-the-FoodDots with color.

| | Where | When | Duration | Distance |
|---|---|---|---|---|
| Exercise | | | | |
| **EXERCISE TOTALS:** | | | | |

# Color in
today's PowerCircles!

Met exercise goal today _____

Days in a row of
Lean Mode journaling _____    _____ lbs.

Met food goal today _____

- free day _____

Glasses of water _____

Su  M  Tu  W  Th  F  Sa    Select Day
of Week

# Lean Mode Food Diary **Daily Page** FOR ____/____/____

| What I ate/drank | Where/When | Quantity | Calories | Fat Grams | Carbs Grams | Fiber Grams | Protein Grams |
|---|---|---|---|---|---|---|---|
| | | | | | | | |
| | | | | | | | |
| | | | | | | | |
| | | | | | | | |
| | | | | | | | |
| | | | | | | | |
| | | | | | | | |
| | | | | | | | |
| | | | | | | | |
| | | | | | | | |
| | | | | | | | |
| | | | | | | | |
| **FOOD TOTALS:** | | | | | | | |

**Color in** the FoodDots above that show healthy eating.
Try to connect-the-FoodDots with color.

| | Where | When | Duration | Distance | |
|---|---|---|---|---|---|
| Exercise | | | | | |
| **EXERCISE TOTALS:** | | | | | |

## Color in
today's PowerCircles!

Met exercise goal today _____

Met food goal today _____

Days in a row of
Lean Mode journaling _____        lbs.

- free day _____

Glasses of water _____

# Fill in Your **Color Code & Goals Page**

Take baby steps! Gradually build better habits by setting realistic goals here.

**NOTES:**

Set up your Goals and Color Code for the WEEK of ____/____/____ thru ____/____/____   Journaling Week # _____

| **DAILY GOALS** (Your choice of sections below)<br>◯ Same as last week | **WEEKLY GOALS**<br>◯ Same as last week | **WEEKLY TAB**<br>Review your PowerCircles at week's end |
|---|---|---|
| **My daily food goal is:** _____ **calories**<br><br>My color for meeting all my daily food goals:<br>(  ) (  ) (  ) (  ) | I'll meet the goal at left at least _____ times per week | Did I meet my weekly goal at left?<br>**YES,** I met my weekly goal!<br>(Color it in) |
| **I'll include these healthy foods each day:**<br>FoodDot Color    Food Group/Item    Amount<br><br>Optional Lean Mode Lite Day | I'll meet the goal at left at least<br>_____ times per week<br>_____ times per week<br>_____ times per week | Did I meet my weekly goal at left?<br>**YES,** I met my weekly goal!<br>(Color it in) |
| **I'll color in a** _____ **- free day**<br>(e.g. sugar-free, pastry-free, soda-free, etc.)<br>in this color in this spot in my PowerCircles: | I'll meet the goal at left at least _____ times per week | Did I meet my weekly goal at left?<br>**YES,** I met my weekly goal!<br>(Color it in) |
| **My daily exercise goal is:**<br><br>My color for meeting my daily exercise goal is: | I'll meet the goal at left at least _____ times per week | Did I meet my weekly goal at left?<br>**YES,** I met my weekly goal!<br>(Color it in) |

My **4WEEK BUBBLE REWARD** for meeting all my weekly goals will be: _____

Su  M  Tu  W  Th  F  Sa    Select Day of Week

# Lean Mode Food Diary **Daily Page**   FOR _____ / _____ / _____

| What I ate/drank | Where/When | Quantity | Calories | Fat Grams | Carbs Grams | Fiber Grams | Protein Grams |
|---|---|---|---|---|---|---|---|
| | | | | | | | |
| | | | | | | | |
| | | | | | | | |
| | | | | | | | |
| | | | | | | | |
| | | | | | | | |
| | | | | | | | |
| | | | | | | | |
| | | | | | | | |
| | | | | | | | |
| | | | | | | | |
| | | | | | | | |
| | | | | | | | |
| | | | | | | | |
| | | | | | | | |
| | | | | | | | |
| **FOOD TOTALS:** | | | | | | | |

**Color in** the FoodDots above that show healthy eating.
Try to connect-the-FoodDots with color.

| | Where | When | Duration | Distance |
|---|---|---|---|---|
| Exercise | | | | |
| **EXERCISE TOTALS:** | | | | |

## Color in
### today's PowerCircles!

Met exercise goal today _____

Days in a row of
Lean Mode journaling _____

lbs.

Met food goal today _____

- free day _____

Glasses of water _____

Su M Tu W Th F Sa **Select Day of Week**

# Lean Mode Food Diary **Daily Page** FOR _____ / _____ / _____

| What I ate/drank | Where/When | Quantity | Calories | Fat Grams | Carbs Grams | Fiber Grams | Protein Grams | |
|---|---|---|---|---|---|---|---|---|
| | | | | | | | | |
| | | | | | | | | |
| | | | | | | | | |
| | | | | | | | | |
| | | | | | | | | |
| | | | | | | | | |
| | | | | | | | | |
| | | | | | | | | |
| | | | | | | | | |
| | | | | | | | | |
| **FOOD TOTALS:** | | | | | | | | |

**Color in** the FoodDots above that show healthy eating.
Try to connect-the-FoodDots with color.

| | Where | When | Duration | Distance |
|---|---|---|---|---|
| Exercise | | | | |
| **EXERCISE TOTALS:** | | | | |

# Color in today's PowerCircles!

Met exercise goal today _____

Met food goal today _____

_____ - free day

Days in a row of Lean Mode journaling _____     lbs.

Glasses of water

Su  M  Tu  W  Th  F  Sa   Select Day of Week

# Lean Mode Food Diary **Daily Page** FOR _____ / ____ / ____

| What I ate/drank | Where/When | Quantity | Calories | Fat Grams | Carbs Grams | Fiber Grams | Protein Grams |
|---|---|---|---|---|---|---|---|
| | | | | | | | |
| | | | | | | | |
| | | | | | | | |
| | | | | | | | |
| | | | | | | | |
| | | | | | | | |
| | | | | | | | |
| | | | | | | | |
| | | | | | | | |
| | | | | | | | |
| | | | | | | | |
| | | | | | | | |
| | | | | | | | |
| | | | | | | | |
| **FOOD TOTALS:** | | | | | | | |

**Color in** the FoodDots above that show healthy eating.
Try to connect-the-FoodDots with color.

| | Where | When | Duration | Distance | | |
|---|---|---|---|---|---|---|
| Exercise | | | | | | |
| **EXERCISE TOTALS:** | | | | | | |

## Color in today's PowerCircles!

Met exercise goal today _____

Days in a row of Lean Mode journaling _____

_____ lbs.

Met food goal today _____

- free day _____

Glasses of water _____

# Lean Mode Food Diary **Daily Page** FOR ___ ___ / ___ ___ / ___ ___

| What I ate/drank | Where/When | Quantity | Calories | Fat Grams | Carbs Grams | Fiber Grams | Protein Grams | |
|---|---|---|---|---|---|---|---|---|
| | | | | | | | | |
| | | | | | | | | |
| | | | | | | | | |
| | | | | | | | | |
| | | | | | | | | |
| | | | | | | | | |
| | | | | | | | | |
| | | | | | | | | |
| | | | | | | | | |
| | | | | | | | | |
| | | | | | | | | |
| | | | | | | | | |
| | | | | | | | | |
| | | | | | | | | |
| | | | | | | | | |
| **FOOD TOTALS:** | | | | | | | | |

**Color in** the FoodDots above that show healthy eating.
Try to connect-the-FoodDots with color.

| | Where | When | Duration | Distance |
|---|---|---|---|---|
| Exercise | | | | |
| **EXERCISE TOTALS:** | | | | |

## Color in today's PowerCircles!

Met exercise goal today ___

Met food goal today ___

Days in a row of Lean Mode journaling ___

___ lbs.

- free day ___

Glasses of water ___

# Lean Mode Food Diary **Daily Page** FOR ___ / ___ / ___

| | What I ate/drank | Where/When | Quantity | Calories | Fat Grams | Carbs Grams | Fiber Grams | Protein Grams |
|---|---|---|---|---|---|---|---|---|
| | | | | | | | | |
| | | | | | | | | |
| | | | | | | | | |
| | | | | | | | | |
| | | | | | | | | |
| | | | | | | | | |
| | | | | | | | | |
| | | | | | | | | |
| | | | | | | | | |
| | | | | | | | | |
| | | | | | | | | |
| | | | | | | | | |
| | | | | | | | | |
| | **FOOD TOTALS:** | | | | | | | |

**Color in** the FoodDots above that show healthy eating.
Try to connect-the-FoodDots with color.

| | Where | When | Duration | Distance |
|---|---|---|---|---|
| Exercise | | | | |
| | **EXERCISE TOTALS:** | | | |

## Color in today's PowerCircles!

Met exercise goal today _____

Days in a row of Lean Mode journaling _____

lbs.

Met food goal today _____

- free day

Glasses of water

# Lean Mode Food Diary **Daily Page** FOR ___ / ___ / ___

| What I ate/drank | Where/When | Quantity | Calories | Fat Grams | Carbs Grams | Fiber Grams | Protein Grams |
|---|---|---|---|---|---|---|---|
|  |  |  |  |  |  |  |  |
|  |  |  |  |  |  |  |  |
|  |  |  |  |  |  |  |  |
|  |  |  |  |  |  |  |  |
|  |  |  |  |  |  |  |  |
|  |  |  |  |  |  |  |  |
|  |  |  |  |  |  |  |  |
|  |  |  |  |  |  |  |  |
|  |  |  |  |  |  |  |  |
| **FOOD TOTALS:** |  |  |  |  |  |  |  |

**Color in** the FoodDots above that show healthy eating.
Try to connect-the-FoodDots with color.

| | Where | When | Duration | Distance |
|---|---|---|---|---|
| Exercise |  |  |  |  |
| **EXERCISE TOTALS:** |  |  |  |  |

# Color in
## today's PowerCircles!

Met exercise goal today ___

Days in a row of Lean Mode journaling ___

___ lbs.

Met food goal today ___

- free day ___

Glasses of water ___

Su M Tu W Th F Sa    Select Day of Week

# Lean Mode Food Diary **Daily Page** FOR ____ / ____ / ____

| | What I ate/drank | Where/When | Quantity | Calories | Fat Grams | Carbs Grams | Fiber Grams | Protein Grams | |
|---|---|---|---|---|---|---|---|---|---|
| | | | | | | | | | |
| | | | | | | | | | |
| | | | | | | | | | |
| | | | | | | | | | |
| | | | | | | | | | |
| | | | | | | | | | |
| | | | | | | | | | |
| | | | | | | | | | |
| | | | | | | | | | |
| | | | | | | | | | |
| | | | | | | | | | |
| | | | | | | | | | |
| | | | | | | | | | |
| | **FOOD TOTALS:** | | | | | | | | |

**Color in** the FoodDots above that show healthy eating.
Try to connect-the-FoodDots with color.

| | Where | When | Duration | Distance | |
|---|---|---|---|---|---|
| Exercise | | | | | |
| **EXERCISE TOTALS:** | | | | | |

## Color in today's PowerCircles!

Met exercise goal today ____

Met food goal today ____

- free day ____

Days in a row of Lean Mode journaling ____

____ lbs.

Glasses of water ____

# Complete Your **4Week Bubble**

Look back over your Weekly Tabs for the past 4 weeks and tally the results.

**4WEEK BUBBLE RECAP:** ___/___/___ thru ___/___/___

| | Start | End | + or – |
|---|---|---|---|
| Weight | | | |
| | | | |
| | | | |
| | | | |

**Yay!** I journaled every day

I journaled _____ days this period,
_____ days in a row this period,
and _____ days in a row to date.

The **REWARD** I gave myself for meeting all my weekly goals this period was:

_____
(Color in your **4WEEK BUBBLE** at right)

○ NO, I didn't meet all my weekly goals, but here's what I need to change to succeed next month:

_____

**YES,** I met ALL my weekly goals!

---

Set up your Goals and Color Code for the WEEK of ___/___/___ thru ___/___/___   Journaling Week # _____

| **DAILY GOALS** (Your choice of sections below) ○ Same as last week | **WEEKLY GOALS** ○ Same as last week | **WEEKLY TAB** Review your PowerCircles at week's end |
|---|---|---|
| **My daily food goal is:** _____ **calories** My color for meeting all my daily food goals: ( ) ( ) ( ) ( ) | I'll meet the goal at left at least _____ times per week | Did I meet my weekly goal at left? **YES,** I met my weekly goal! (Color it in) |
| **I'll include these healthy foods each day:** FoodDot Color    Food Group/Item    Amount *Optional Lean Mode Lite Day* | I'll meet the goal at left at least _____ times per week _____ times per week _____ times per week | Did I meet my weekly goal at left? **YES,** I met my weekly goal! (Color it in) |
| **I'll color in a** _____ **- free day** (e.g. sugar-free, pastry-free, soda-free, etc.) in this color in this spot in my PowerCircles: | I'll meet the goal at left at least _____ times per week | Did I meet my weekly goal at left? **YES,** I met my weekly goal! (Color it in) |
| **My daily exercise goal is:** _____ My color for meeting my daily exercise goal is: | I'll meet the goal at left at least _____ times per week | Did I meet my weekly goal at left? **YES,** I met my weekly goal! (Color it in) |

My **4WEEK BUBBLE REWARD** for meeting all my weekly goals will be: _____

Su M Tu W Th F Sa   Select Day of Week

# Lean Mode Food Diary **Daily Page**  FOR ____ / ____ / ____

| What I ate/drank | Where/When | Quantity | Calories | Fat Grams | Carbs Grams | Fiber Grams | Protein Grams |
|---|---|---|---|---|---|---|---|
| | | | | | | | |
| | | | | | | | |
| | | | | | | | |
| | | | | | | | |
| | | | | | | | |
| | | | | | | | |
| | | | | | | | |
| | | | | | | | |
| | | | | | | | |
| | | | | | | | |
| | | | | | | | |
| | | | | | | | |
| | | | | | | | |
| **FOOD TOTALS:** | | | | | | | |

**Color in** the FoodDots above that show healthy eating.
Try to connect-the-FoodDots with color.

| | Where | When | Duration | Distance |
|---|---|---|---|---|
| Exercise | | | | |
| **EXERCISE TOTALS:** | | | | |

## Color in today's PowerCircles!

Met exercise goal today ____

Days in a row of Lean Mode journaling ____        lbs.

Met food goal today ____

- free day ____

Glasses of water ____

(Su) (M) (Tu) (W) (Th) (F) (Sa)  **Select Day of Week**

# Lean Mode Food Diary **Daily Page** FOR _____ / _____ / _____

| What I ate/drank | Where/When | Quantity | Calories | Fat Grams | Carbs Grams | Fiber Grams | Protein Grams |
|---|---|---|---|---|---|---|---|
|  |  |  |  |  |  |  |  |
|  |  |  |  |  |  |  |  |
|  |  |  |  |  |  |  |  |
|  |  |  |  |  |  |  |  |
|  |  |  |  |  |  |  |  |
|  |  |  |  |  |  |  |  |
|  |  |  |  |  |  |  |  |
|  |  |  |  |  |  |  |  |
|  |  |  |  |  |  |  |  |
|  |  |  |  |  |  |  |  |
|  |  |  |  |  |  |  |  |
| **FOOD TOTALS:** |  |  |  |  |  |  |  |

**Color in** the FoodDots above that show healthy eating.
Try to connect-the-FoodDots with color.

| | Where | When | Duration | Distance |
|---|---|---|---|---|
| Exercise |  |  |  |  |
| **EXERCISE TOTALS:** |  |  |  |  |

# Color in
## today's PowerCircles!

Met exercise goal today _____

Days in a row of
Lean Mode journaling _____

lbs.

Met food goal today _____

- free day _____

Glasses of water _____

# Lean Mode Food Diary **Daily Page** FOR _____ / _____ / _____

| | What I ate/drank | Where/When | Quantity | Calories | Fat Grams | Carbs Grams | Fiber Grams | Protein Grams | |
|---|---|---|---|---|---|---|---|---|---|
| | | | | | | | | | |
| | | | | | | | | | |
| | | | | | | | | | |
| | | | | | | | | | |
| | | | | | | | | | |
| | | | | | | | | | |
| | | | | | | | | | |
| | | | | | | | | | |
| | | | | | | | | | |
| | | | | | | | | | |
| | | | | | | | | | |
| | | | | | | | | | |
| | | | | | | | | | |
| | | | | | | | | | |
| | | | | | | | | | |
| | **FOOD TOTALS:** | | | | | | | | |

**Color in** the FoodDots above that show healthy eating.
Try to connect-the-FoodDots with color.

| | | Where | When | Duration | Distance | |
|---|---|---|---|---|---|---|
| Exercise | | | | | | |
| | | | | | | |
| | **EXERCISE TOTALS:** | | | | | |

## Color in today's PowerCircles!

Met exercise goal today _____

Days in a row of
Lean Mode journaling _____

_____ lbs.

Met food goal today _____

- free day _____

Glasses of water _____

# Lean Mode Food Diary **Daily Page** FOR _____ / _____ / _____

| What I ate/drank | Where/When | Quantity | Calories | Fat Grams | Carbs Grams | Fiber Grams | Protein Grams | |
|---|---|---|---|---|---|---|---|---|
| | | | | | | | | |
| | | | | | | | | |
| | | | | | | | | |
| | | | | | | | | |
| | | | | | | | | |
| | | | | | | | | |
| | | | | | | | | |
| | | | | | | | | |
| | | | | | | | | |
| | | | | | | | | |
| | | | | | | | | |
| | | | | | | | | |
| **FOOD TOTALS:** | | | | | | | | |

**Color in** the FoodDots above that show healthy eating.
Try to connect-the-FoodDots with color.

| | Where | When | Duration | Distance |
|---|---|---|---|---|
| Exercise | | | | |
| **EXERCISE TOTALS:** | | | | |

# Color in
## today's PowerCircles!

Met exercise goal today _____

Days in a row of
Lean Mode journaling _____

lbs.

Met food goal today _____

- free day _____

Glasses of water _____

# Lean Mode Food Diary **Daily Page** FOR ____ / ____ / ____

| | What I ate/drank | Where/When | Quantity | Calories | Fat Grams | Carbs Grams | Fiber Grams | Protein Grams |
|---|---|---|---|---|---|---|---|---|
| | | | | | | | | |
| | | | | | | | | |
| | | | | | | | | |
| | | | | | | | | |
| | | | | | | | | |
| | | | | | | | | |
| | | | | | | | | |
| | | | | | | | | |
| | | | | | | | | |
| | | | | | | | | |
| | | | | | | | | |
| | | | | | | | | |
| | | | | | | | | |
| | | | | | | | | |
| | | | | | | | | |
| | **FOOD TOTALS:** | | | | | | | |

**Color in** the FoodDots above that show healthy eating.
Try to connect-the-FoodDots with color.

| | Where | When | Duration | Distance |
|---|---|---|---|---|
| Exercise | | | | |
| **EXERCISE TOTALS:** | | | | |

## Color in today's PowerCircles!

Met exercise goal today _____

Met food goal today _____

- free day _____

Days in a row of Lean Mode journaling _____

____ lbs.

Glasses of water _____

Su  M  Tu  W  Th  F  Sa  Select Day
of Week

# Lean Mode Food Diary **Daily Page** FOR ____ / ____ / ____

| What I ate/drank | Where/When | Quantity | Calories | Fat Grams | Carbs Grams | Fiber Grams | Protein Grams | |
|---|---|---|---|---|---|---|---|---|
| | | | | | | | | |
| | | | | | | | | |
| | | | | | | | | |
| | | | | | | | | |
| | | | | | | | | |
| | | | | | | | | |
| | | | | | | | | |
| | | | | | | | | |
| | | | | | | | | |
| | | | | | | | | |
| | | | | | | | | |
| | | | | | | | | |

**FOOD TOTALS:**

**Color in** the FoodDots above that show healthy eating.
Try to connect-the-FoodDots with color.

| | Where | When | Duration | Distance |
|---|---|---|---|---|
| Exercise | | | | |

**EXERCISE TOTALS:**

# Color in
## today's PowerCircles!

Met exercise goal today ____

Met food goal today ____

____ - free day

Days in a row of
Lean Mode journaling ____

____ lbs.

Glasses of water ____

Su M Tu W Th F Sa   Select Day of Week

# Lean Mode Food Diary **Daily Page** FOR _____ / _____ / _____

| What I ate/drank | Where/When | Quantity | Calories | Fat Grams | Carbs Grams | Fiber Grams | Protein Grams |
|---|---|---|---|---|---|---|---|
| | | | | | | | |
| | | | | | | | |
| | | | | | | | |
| | | | | | | | |
| | | | | | | | |
| | | | | | | | |
| | | | | | | | |
| | | | | | | | |
| | | | | | | | |
| | | | | | | | |
| **FOOD TOTALS:** | | | | | | | |

**Color in** the FoodDots above that show healthy eating. Try to connect-the-FoodDots with color.

| | Where | When | Duration | Distance |
|---|---|---|---|---|
| Exercise | | | | |
| | | | | |
| **EXERCISE TOTALS:** | | | | |

## Color in today's PowerCircles!

Met exercise goal today _____

Met food goal today _____

- free day _____

Days in a row of Lean Mode journaling _____

lbs.

Glasses of water _____

# Fill in Your **Color Code & Goals Page**

Take baby steps! Gradually build better habits by setting realistic goals here.

**NOTES:**

Set up your Goals and Color Code for the WEEK of __ __/__ __/__ __ thru __ __/__ __/__ __   Journaling Week # __ __ __

| **DAILY GOALS** (Your choice of sections below) | **WEEKLY GOALS** | **WEEKLY TAB** |
|---|---|---|
| ⚪ Same as last week | ⚪ Same as last week | Review your PowerCircles at week's end |
| **My daily food goal is:** ............ **calories**<br><br>My color for meeting all my daily food goals:<br>............ ( )<br>............ ( )<br>............ ( )<br>............ ( ) | I'll meet the goal at left at least ......... times per week | Did I meet my weekly goal at left?<br><br>**YES,** I met my weekly goal!<br>(Color it in) |
| **I'll include these healthy foods each day:**<br><br>FoodDot Color    Food Group/Item    Amount<br><br>Optional Lean Mode Lite Day | I'll meet the goal at left at least<br><br>......... times per week<br>......... times per week<br>......... times per week | Did I meet my weekly goal at left?<br><br>**YES,** I met my weekly goal!<br>(Color it in) |
| **I'll color in a** ............ **- free day**<br>(e.g. sugar-free, pastry-free, soda-free, etc.)<br><br>in this color in this spot in my PowerCircles: | I'll meet the goal at left at least ......... times per week | Did I meet my weekly goal at left?<br><br>**YES,** I met my weekly goal!<br>(Color it in) |
| **My daily exercise goal is:** ............<br><br>My color for meeting my daily exercise goal is: | I'll meet the goal at left at least ......... times per week | Did I meet my weekly goal at left?<br><br>**YES,** I met my weekly goal!<br>(Color it in) |

My **4WEEK BUBBLE REWARD** for meeting all my weekly goals will be: _____

Su  M  Tu  W  Th  F  Sa    Select Day
of Week

# Lean Mode Food Diary **Daily Page**  FOR _____ / _____ / _____

| What I ate/drank | Where/When | Quantity | Calories | Fat Grams | Carbs Grams | Fiber Grams | Protein Grams |
|---|---|---|---|---|---|---|---|
|  |  |  |  |  |  |  |  |
|  |  |  |  |  |  |  |  |
|  |  |  |  |  |  |  |  |
|  |  |  |  |  |  |  |  |
|  |  |  |  |  |  |  |  |
|  |  |  |  |  |  |  |  |
|  |  |  |  |  |  |  |  |
|  |  |  |  |  |  |  |  |
|  |  |  |  |  |  |  |  |
|  |  |  |  |  |  |  |  |
|  |  |  |  |  |  |  |  |
| **FOOD TOTALS:** |  |  |  |  |  |  |  |

**Color in** the FoodDots above that show healthy eating.
Try to connect-the-FoodDots with color.

| | Where | When | Duration | Distance | | |
|---|---|---|---|---|---|---|
| Exercise |  |  |  |  |  |  |
| **EXERCISE TOTALS:** |  |  |  |  |  |  |

## Color in
today's PowerCircles!

Met exercise goal today _____

Days in a row of
Lean Mode journaling _____

lbs.

Met food goal today _____

- free day _____

Glasses of water _____

# Lean Mode Food Diary **Daily Page** FOR _____ / _____ / _____

| What I ate/drank | | Where/When | Quantity | Calories | Fat Grams | Carbs Grams | Fiber Grams | Protein Grams | |
|---|---|---|---|---|---|---|---|---|---|
| | | | | | | | | | |
| | | | | | | | | | |
| | | | | | | | | | |
| | | | | | | | | | |
| | | | | | | | | | |
| | | | | | | | | | |
| | | | | | | | | | |
| | | | | | | | | | |
| | | | | | | | | | |
| | | | | | | | | | |
| **FOOD TOTALS:** | | | | | | | | | |

**Color in** the FoodDots above that show healthy eating.
Try to connect-the-FoodDots with color.

| | Where | When | Duration | Distance | |
|---|---|---|---|---|---|
| Exercise | | | | | |
| **EXERCISE TOTALS:** | | | | | |

# Color in
## today's PowerCircles!

Met exercise goal today _____

Met food goal today _____

- free day _____

Days in a row of
Lean Mode journaling _____        lbs.        Glasses of water _____

Su  M  Tu  W  Th  F  Sa   Select Day of Week

# Lean Mode Food Diary **Daily Page**  FOR  _____ / _____ / _____

| What I ate/drank | Where/When | Quantity | Calories | Fat Grams | Carbs Grams | Fiber Grams | Protein Grams | |
|---|---|---|---|---|---|---|---|---|
| | | | | | | | | |
| | | | | | | | | |
| | | | | | | | | |
| | | | | | | | | |
| | | | | | | | | |
| | | | | | | | | |
| | | | | | | | | |
| | | | | | | | | |
| | | | | | | | | |
| | | | | | | | | |
| | | | | | | | | |
| | | | | | | | | |
| | | | | | | | | |
| **FOOD TOTALS:** | | | | | | | | |

**Color in** the FoodDots above that show healthy eating.
Try to connect-the-FoodDots with color.

| | Where | When | Duration | Distance | |
|---|---|---|---|---|---|
| Exercise | | | | | |
| **EXERCISE TOTALS:** | | | | | |

# Color in
## today's PowerCircles!

Met exercise goal today _____

Days in a row of
Lean Mode journaling _____

lbs.

Met food goal today _____

- free day _____

Glasses of water _____

Su M Tu W Th F Sa **Select Day of Week**

# Lean Mode Food Diary **Daily Page** FOR _____ / _____ / _____

| What I ate/drank | Where/When | Quantity | Calories | Fat Grams | Carbs Grams | Fiber Grams | Protein Grams |
|---|---|---|---|---|---|---|---|
| | | | | | | | |
| | | | | | | | |
| | | | | | | | |
| | | | | | | | |
| | | | | | | | |
| | | | | | | | |
| | | | | | | | |
| | | | | | | | |
| | | | | | | | |
| | | | | | | | |
| | | | | | | | |
| | | | | | | | |
| | | | | | | | |
| **FOOD TOTALS:** | | | | | | | |

**Color in** the FoodDots above that show healthy eating.
Try to connect-the-FoodDots with color.

| | Where | When | Duration | Distance |
|---|---|---|---|---|
| Exercise | | | | |
| **EXERCISE TOTALS:** | | | | |

## Color in today's PowerCircles!

Met exercise goal today _____

Days in a row of
Lean Mode journaling _____            lbs.

Met food goal today _____

- free day _____

Glasses of water _____

Su  M  Tu  W  Th  F  Sa    Select Day of Week

# Lean Mode Food Diary **Daily Page** FOR ____/____/____

| | What I ate/drank | Where/When | Quantity | Calories | Fat Grams | Carbs Grams | Fiber Grams | Protein Grams |
|---|---|---|---|---|---|---|---|---|
| | | | | | | | | |
| | | | | | | | | |
| | | | | | | | | |
| | | | | | | | | |
| | | | | | | | | |
| | | | | | | | | |
| | | | | | | | | |
| | | | | | | | | |
| | | | | | | | | |
| | | | | | | | | |
| | | | | | | | | |
| | | | | | | | | |
| | | | | | | | | |
| | | | | | | | | |
| | | | | | | | | |
| | | | | | | | | |
| | **FOOD TOTALS:** | | | | | | | |

**Color in** the FoodDots above that show healthy eating.
Try to connect-the-FoodDots with color.

| | Where | When | Duration | Distance | |
|---|---|---|---|---|---|
| Exercise | | | | | |
| | | | | | |
| **EXERCISE TOTALS:** | | | | | |

# Color in
## today's PowerCircles!

Met exercise goal today ............................................

Days in a row of
Lean Mode journaling ..............................  lbs.

Met food goal today ............................................

- free day

Glasses of water

Su  M  Tu  W  Th  F  Sa  Select Day
of Week

# Lean Mode Food Diary **Daily Page** FOR _____ / _____ / _____

| What I ate/drank | Where/When | Quantity | Calories | Fat Grams | Carbs Grams | Fiber Grams | Protein Grams | |
|---|---|---|---|---|---|---|---|---|
| | | | | | | | | |
| | | | | | | | | |
| | | | | | | | | |
| | | | | | | | | |
| | | | | | | | | |
| | | | | | | | | |
| | | | | | | | | |
| | | | | | | | | |
| | | | | | | | | |
| | | | | | | | | |
| | | | | | | | | |
| | | | | | | | | |
| | | | | | | | | |
| **FOOD TOTALS:** | | | | | | | | |

**Color in** the FoodDots above that show healthy eating.
Try to connect-the-FoodDots with color.

| | Where | When | Duration | Distance |
|---|---|---|---|---|
| Exercise | | | | |
| | | | | |
| **EXERCISE TOTALS:** | | | | |

## Color in today's PowerCircles!

Met exercise goal today _____

Days in a row of Lean Mode journaling _____

lbs.

Met food goal today _____

- free day _____

Glasses of water _____

# Lean Mode Food Diary **Daily Page** FOR _____ / _____ / _____

| What I ate/drank | Where/When | Quantity | Calories | Fat Grams | Carbs Grams | Fiber Grams | Protein Grams | |
|---|---|---|---|---|---|---|---|---|
| | | | | | | | | |
| | | | | | | | | |
| | | | | | | | | |
| | | | | | | | | |
| | | | | | | | | |
| | | | | | | | | |
| | | | | | | | | |
| | | | | | | | | |
| | | | | | | | | |
| | | | | | | | | |
| | | | | | | | | |
| | | | | | | | | |
| **FOOD TOTALS:** | | | | | | | | |

**Color in** the FoodDots above that show healthy eating.
Try to connect-the-FoodDots with color.

| | Where | When | Duration | Distance |
|---|---|---|---|---|
| Exercise | | | | |
| **EXERCISE TOTALS:** | | | | |

# Color in
## today's PowerCircles!

Met exercise goal today _____

Days in a row of
Lean Mode journaling _____

lbs.

Met food goal today _____

- free day _____

Glasses of water _____

# Fill in Your **Color Code & Goals Page**

Take baby steps! Gradually build better habits by setting realistic goals here.

**NOTES:**

Set up your Goals and Color Code for the WEEK of ___ / ___ / ___ thru ___ / ___ / ___   Journaling Week # _____

| **DAILY GOALS** (Your choice of sections below) ⭕ Same as last week | **WEEKLY GOALS** ⭕ Same as last week | **WEEKLY TAB** Review your PowerCircles at week's end |
|---|---|---|
| **My daily food goal is:** _____ **calories** My color for meeting all my daily food goals: ( ) ( ) ( ) ( ) | I'll meet the goal at left at least _____ times per week | Did I meet my weekly goal at left? **YES,** I met my weekly goal! (Color it in) |
| **I'll include these healthy foods each day:** FoodDot Color    Food Group/Item    Amount _Optional Lean Mode Lite Day_ | I'll meet the goal at left at least _____ times per week _____ times per week _____ times per week | Did I meet my weekly goal at left? **YES,** I met my weekly goal! (Color it in) |
| **I'll color in a** _____ **- free day** (e.g. sugar-free, pastry-free, soda-free, etc.) in this color in this spot in my PowerCircles: | I'll meet the goal at left at least _____ times per week | Did I meet my weekly goal at left? **YES,** I met my weekly goal! (Color it in) |
| **My daily exercise goal is:** _____ My color for meeting my daily exercise goal is: | I'll meet the goal at left at least _____ times per week | Did I meet my weekly goal at left? **YES,** I met my weekly goal! (Color it in) |

My **4WEEK BUBBLE REWARD** for meeting all my weekly goals will be: _____

# Lean Mode Food Diary **Daily Page** FOR ___ / ___ / ___

| | What I ate/drank | Where/When | Quantity | Calories | Fat Grams | Carbs Grams | Fiber Grams | Protein Grams | |
|---|---|---|---|---|---|---|---|---|---|
| | | | | | | | | | |
| | | | | | | | | | |
| | | | | | | | | | |
| | | | | | | | | | |
| | | | | | | | | | |
| | | | | | | | | | |
| | | | | | | | | | |
| | | | | | | | | | |
| | | | | | | | | | |
| | | | | | | | | | |
| | | | | | | | | | |
| | | | | | | | | | |
| | | | | | | | | | |
| | | | | | | | | | |
| | **FOOD TOTALS:** | | | | | | | | |

**Color in** the FoodDots above that show healthy eating.
Try to connect-the-FoodDots with color.

| | Where | When | Duration | Distance | | |
|---|---|---|---|---|---|---|
| Exercise | | | | | | |
| | | | | | | |
| **EXERCISE TOTALS:** | | | | | | |

# Color in
## today's PowerCircles!

Met exercise goal today ___

Days in a row of Lean Mode journaling ___

lbs.

Met food goal today ___

- free day ___

Glasses of water ___

Su M Tu W Th F Sa  Select Day of Week

# Lean Mode Food Diary **Daily Page** FOR ____ / ____ / ____

| What I ate/drank | Where/When | Quantity | Calories | Fat Grams | Carbs Grams | Fiber Grams | Protein Grams | |
|---|---|---|---|---|---|---|---|---|
| | | | | | | | | |
| | | | | | | | | |
| | | | | | | | | |
| | | | | | | | | |
| | | | | | | | | |
| | | | | | | | | |
| | | | | | | | | |
| | | | | | | | | |
| | | | | | | | | |
| | | | | | | | | |
| **FOOD TOTALS:** | | | | | | | | |

**Color in** the FoodDots above that show healthy eating.
Try to connect-the-FoodDots with color.

| | Where | When | Duration | Distance |
|---|---|---|---|---|
| Exercise | | | | |
| | | | | |
| **EXERCISE TOTALS:** | | | | |

## Color in today's PowerCircles!

Met exercise goal today _____

Met food goal today _____

Days in a row of Lean Mode journaling _____

lbs.

- free day _____

Glasses of water _____

Su  M  Tu  W  Th  F  Sa   Select Day
of Week

# Lean Mode Food Diary **Daily Page** FOR _____ / _____ / _____

| What I ate/drank | Where/When | Quantity | Calories | Fat Grams | Carbs Grams | Fiber Grams | Protein Grams | |
|---|---|---|---|---|---|---|---|---|
| | | | | | | | | |
| | | | | | | | | |
| | | | | | | | | |
| | | | | | | | | |
| | | | | | | | | |
| | | | | | | | | |
| | | | | | | | | |
| | | | | | | | | |
| | | | | | | | | |
| | | | | | | | | |
| | | | | | | | | |
| | | | | | | | | |
| | | | | | | | | |
| **FOOD TOTALS:** | | | | | | | | |

**Color in** the FoodDots above that show healthy eating.
Try to connect-the-FoodDots with color.

| | Where | When | Duration | Distance | |
|---|---|---|---|---|---|
| Exercise | | | | | |
| **EXERCISE TOTALS:** | | | | | |

## Color in
today's PowerCircles!

Met exercise goal today _____

Met food goal today _____

- free day

Days in a row of
Lean Mode journaling _____    lbs.    Glasses of water

Su M Tu W Th F Sa **Select Day of Week**

# Lean Mode Food Diary **Daily Page** FOR _____ / _____ / _____

| | What I ate/drank | Where/When | Quantity | Calories | Fat Grams | Carbs Grams | Fiber Grams | Protein Grams | |
|---|---|---|---|---|---|---|---|---|---|
| | | | | | | | | | |
| | | | | | | | | | |
| | | | | | | | | | |
| | | | | | | | | | |
| | | | | | | | | | |
| | | | | | | | | | |
| | | | | | | | | | |
| | | | | | | | | | |
| | | | | | | | | | |
| | | | | | | | | | |
| | | | | | | | | | |
| | | | | | | | | | |
| | | | | | | | | | |
| | | | | | | | | | |
| | **FOOD TOTALS:** | | | | | | | | |

**Color in** the FoodDots above that show healthy eating.
Try to connect-the-FoodDots with color.

| | | Where | When | Duration | Distance | |
|---|---|---|---|---|---|---|
| Exercise | | | | | | |
| | **EXERCISE TOTALS:** | | | | | |

# Color in
## today's PowerCircles!

Met exercise goal today _____

Met food goal today _____

- free day _____

Days in a row of
Lean Mode journaling _____

lbs.

Glasses of water _____

Su M Tu W Th F Sa    Select Day of Week

# Lean Mode Food Diary **Daily Page** FOR _____ / _____ / _____

| | What I ate/drank | Where/When | Quantity | Calories | Fat Grams | Carbs Grams | Fiber Grams | Protein Grams |
|---|---|---|---|---|---|---|---|---|
| | | | | | | | | |
| | | | | | | | | |
| | | | | | | | | |
| | | | | | | | | |
| | | | | | | | | |
| | | | | | | | | |
| | | | | | | | | |
| | | | | | | | | |
| | | | | | | | | |
| | | | | | | | | |
| | | | | | | | | |
| | | | | | | | | |
| | **FOOD TOTALS:** | | | | | | | |

**Color in** the FoodDots above that show healthy eating.
Try to connect-the-FoodDots with color.

| | | Where | When | Duration | Distance |
|---|---|---|---|---|---|
| Exercise | | | | | |
| | **EXERCISE TOTALS:** | | | | |

# Color in
## today's PowerCircles!

Met exercise goal today _____

Met food goal today _____

- free day _____

Days in a row of Lean Mode journaling _____    lbs.    Glasses of water _____

# Lean Mode Food Diary **Daily Page** FOR _____ / ___ / _____

| What I ate/drank | Where/When | Quantity | Calories | Fat Grams | Carbs Grams | Fiber Grams | Protein Grams |
|---|---|---|---|---|---|---|---|
| | | | | | | | |
| | | | | | | | |
| | | | | | | | |
| | | | | | | | |
| | | | | | | | |
| | | | | | | | |
| | | | | | | | |
| | | | | | | | |
| | | | | | | | |
| | | | | | | | |
| **FOOD TOTALS:** | | | | | | | |

**Color in** the FoodDots above that show healthy eating.
Try to connect-the-FoodDots with color.

| | Where | When | Duration | Distance |
|---|---|---|---|---|
| Exercise | | | | |
| **EXERCISE TOTALS:** | | | | |

## Color in today's PowerCircles!

Met exercise goal today _____

Days in a row of Lean Mode journaling _____

_____ lbs.

Met food goal today _____

- free day _____

Glasses of water _____

Su M Tu W Th F Sa    Select Day of Week

# Lean Mode Food Diary **Daily Page** FOR _____ / _____ / _____

| What I ate/drank | Where/When | Quantity | Calories | Fat Grams | Carbs Grams | Fiber Grams | Protein Grams | |
|---|---|---|---|---|---|---|---|---|
| | | | | | | | | |
| | | | | | | | | |
| | | | | | | | | |
| | | | | | | | | |
| | | | | | | | | |
| | | | | | | | | |
| | | | | | | | | |
| | | | | | | | | |
| | | | | | | | | |
| | | | | | | | | |
| | | | | | | | | |
| | | | | | | | | |
| | | | | | | | | |
| **FOOD TOTALS:** | | | | | | | | |

**Color in** the FoodDots above that show healthy eating.
Try to connect-the-FoodDots with color.

| | Where | When | Duration | Distance | | |
|---|---|---|---|---|---|---|
| Exercise | | | | | | |
| **EXERCISE TOTALS:** | | | | | | |

## Color in today's PowerCircles!

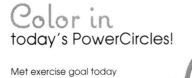

Met exercise goal today _____

Days in a row of Lean Mode journaling _____

lbs.

Met food goal today _____

- free day _____

Glasses of water _____

# Fill in Your **Color Code & Goals Page**

Take baby steps! Gradually build better habits by setting realistic goals here.

**NOTES:**

Set up your Goals and Color Code for the WEEK of ___/___/___ thru ___/___/___    Journaling Week # _____

| **DAILY GOALS** (Your choice of sections below) ⭕ Same as last week | **WEEKLY GOALS** ⭕ Same as last week | **WEEKLY TAB** Review your PowerCircles at week's end |
|---|---|---|
| **My daily food goal is:** _____ **calories** My color for meeting all my daily food goals: ( ) ( ) ( ) ( ) | I'll meet the goal at left at least _____ times per week | Did I meet my weekly goal at left? **YES,** I met my weekly goal! (Color it in) |
| **I'll include these healthy foods each day:** FoodDot Color    Food Group/Item    Amount _Optional Lean Mode Lite Day_ | I'll meet the goal at left at least _____ times per week _____ times per week _____ times per week | Did I meet my weekly goal at left? **YES,** I met my weekly goal! (Color it in) |
| **I'll color in a** _____ **- free day** (e.g. sugar-free, pastry-free, soda-free, etc.) in this color in this spot in my PowerCircles: | I'll meet the goal at left at least _____ times per week | Did I meet my weekly goal at left? **YES,** I met my weekly goal! (Color it in) |
| **My daily exercise goal is:** _____ My color for meeting my daily exercise goal is: | I'll meet the goal at left at least _____ times per week | Did I meet my weekly goal at left? **YES,** I met my weekly goal! (Color it in) |

My **4WEEK BUBBLE REWARD** for meeting all my weekly goals will be: _____

Su  M  Tu  W  Th  F  Sa  Select Day of Week

# Lean Mode Food Diary **Daily Page** FOR ____ / ____ / ____

| What I ate/drank | Where/When | Quantity | Calories | Fat Grams | Carbs Grams | Fiber Grams | Protein Grams |
|---|---|---|---|---|---|---|---|
| | | | | | | | |
| | | | | | | | |
| | | | | | | | |
| | | | | | | | |
| | | | | | | | |
| | | | | | | | |
| | | | | | | | |
| | | | | | | | |
| | | | | | | | |
| | | | | | | | |
| | | | | | | | |
| | | | | | | | |
| | | | | | | | |
| | | | | | | | |
| | | | | | | | |
| **FOOD TOTALS:** | | | | | | | |

**Color in** the FoodDots above that show healthy eating.
Try to connect-the-FoodDots with color.

| | Where | When | Duration | Distance |
|---|---|---|---|---|
| Exercise | | | | |
| **EXERCISE TOTALS:** | | | | |

# Color in
## today's PowerCircles!

Met exercise goal today _____

Met food goal today _____

- free day

Days in a row of Lean Mode journaling _____

lbs.

Glasses of water

# Lean Mode Food Diary **Daily Page**   FOR _____ / _____ / _____

| | What I ate/drank | Where/When | Quantity | Calories | Fat Grams | Carbs Grams | Fiber Grams | Protein Grams | |
|---|---|---|---|---|---|---|---|---|---|
| | | | | | | | | | |
| | | | | | | | | | |
| | | | | | | | | | |
| | | | | | | | | | |
| | | | | | | | | | |
| | | | | | | | | | |
| | | | | | | | | | |
| | | | | | | | | | |
| | | | | | | | | | |
| | | | | | | | | | |
| | | | | | | | | | |
| | | | | | | | | | |
| | | | | | | | | | |

**FOOD TOTALS:**

**Color in** the FoodDots above that show healthy eating.
Try to connect-the-FoodDots with color.

| | | Where | When | Duration | Distance | |
|---|---|---|---|---|---|---|
| Exercise | | | | | | |

**EXERCISE TOTALS:**

## Color in
## today's PowerCircles!

Met exercise goal today _____

Days in a row of
Lean Mode journaling _____

_____ lbs.

Met food goal today _____

- free day _____

Glasses of water _____

# Lean Mode Food Diary **Daily Page** FOR ____ / ____ / ____

| | What I ate/drank | Where/When | Quantity | Calories | Fat Grams | Carbs Grams | Fiber Grams | Protein Grams |
|---|---|---|---|---|---|---|---|---|
| | | | | | | | | |
| | | | | | | | | |
| | | | | | | | | |
| | | | | | | | | |
| | | | | | | | | |
| | | | | | | | | |
| | | | | | | | | |
| | | | | | | | | |
| | | | | | | | | |
| | | | | | | | | |
| | | | | | | | | |
| | | | | | | | | |
| | **FOOD TOTALS:** | | | | | | | |

**Color in** the FoodDots above that show healthy eating.
Try to connect-the-FoodDots with color.

| | Where | When | Duration | Distance |
|---|---|---|---|---|
| Exercise | | | | |
| **EXERCISE TOTALS:** | | | | |

## Color in today's PowerCircles!

Met exercise goal today ____

Days in a row of Lean Mode journaling ____    lbs.

Met food goal today ____

- free day ____

Glasses of water ____

# Lean Mode Food Diary **Daily Page** FOR ____ / ____ / ____

| What I ate/drank | Where/When | Quantity | Calories | Fat Grams | Carbs Grams | Fiber Grams | Protein Grams |
|---|---|---|---|---|---|---|---|
| | | | | | | | |

**FOOD TOTALS:**

**Color in** the FoodDots above that show healthy eating.
Try to connect-the-FoodDots with color.

| | Where | When | Duration | Distance |
|---|---|---|---|---|
| Exercise | | | | |

**EXERCISE TOTALS:**

# Color in today's PowerCircles!

Met exercise goal today

Met food goal today

- free day

Days in a row of Lean Mode journaling

lbs.

Glasses of water

Su  M  Tu  W  Th  F  Sa   Select Day of Week

# Lean Mode Food Diary **Daily Page** FOR _____ / ____ / _____

| What I ate/drank | Where/When | Quantity | Calories | Fat Grams | Carbs Grams | Fiber Grams | Protein Grams | |
|---|---|---|---|---|---|---|---|---|
| | | | | | | | | |
| | | | | | | | | |
| | | | | | | | | |
| | | | | | | | | |
| | | | | | | | | |
| | | | | | | | | |
| | | | | | | | | |
| | | | | | | | | |
| | | | | | | | | |
| | | | | | | | | |
| | | | | | | | | |
| | | | | | | | | |
| | | | | | | | | |
| **FOOD TOTALS:** | | | | | | | | |

**Color in** the FoodDots above that show healthy eating.
Try to connect-the-FoodDots with color.

| | Where | When | Duration | Distance | |
|---|---|---|---|---|---|
| Exercise | | | | | |
| **EXERCISE TOTALS:** | | | | | |

## Color in today's PowerCircles!

Met exercise goal today ........................................

Met food goal today ........................................

- free day

Days in a row of Lean Mode journaling ........................    ____ lbs.

Glasses of water

# Lean Mode Food Diary **Daily Page** FOR _____ / _____ / _____

| What I ate/drank | Where/When | Quantity | Calories | Fat Grams | Carbs Grams | Fiber Grams | Protein Grams | |
|---|---|---|---|---|---|---|---|---|
| | | | | | | | | |
| | | | | | | | | |
| | | | | | | | | |
| | | | | | | | | |
| | | | | | | | | |
| | | | | | | | | |
| | | | | | | | | |
| | | | | | | | | |
| | | | | | | | | |
| | | | | | | | | |
| | | | | | | | | |
| | | | | | | | | |
| | | | | | | | | |
| **FOOD TOTALS:** | | | | | | | | |

**Color in** the FoodDots above that show healthy eating.
Try to connect-the-FoodDots with color.

| | Where | When | Duration | Distance | |
|---|---|---|---|---|---|
| Exercise | | | | | |
| | | | | | |
| **EXERCISE TOTALS:** | | | | | |

## Color in today's PowerCircles!

Met exercise goal today _____

Met food goal today _____

- free day _____

Days in a row of
Lean Mode journaling _____      lbs.

Glasses of water _____

Su M Tu W Th F Sa  Select Day of Week

# Lean Mode Food Diary **Daily Page** FOR ___/___/___

| What I ate/drank | Where/When | Quantity | Calories | Fat Grams | Carbs Grams | Fiber Grams | Protein Grams |
|---|---|---|---|---|---|---|---|
| | | | | | | | |
| | | | | | | | |
| | | | | | | | |
| | | | | | | | |
| | | | | | | | |
| | | | | | | | |
| | | | | | | | |
| | | | | | | | |
| | | | | | | | |
| | | | | | | | |
| | | | | | | | |
| | | | | | | | |
| | | | | | | | |
| | | | | | | | |
| FOOD TOTALS: | | | | | | | |

**Color in** the FoodDots above that show healthy eating.
Try to connect-the-FoodDots with color.

| | Where | When | Duration | Distance |
|---|---|---|---|---|
| Exercise | | | | |
| EXERCISE TOTALS: | | | | |

## Color in today's PowerCircles!

Met exercise goal today ___

Met food goal today ___

Days in a row of Lean Mode journaling ___

lbs. ___

- free day ___

Glasses of water ___

# Complete Your **4Week Bubble**

Look back over your Weekly Tabs for the past 4 weeks and tally the results.

**4WEEK BUBBLE RECAP:** ___/___/___thru___/___/___

|  | Start | End | + or – |
|---|---|---|---|
| Weight |  |  |  |
|  |  |  |  |
|  |  |  |  |

**Yay!** I journaled every day

I journaled _____ days this period,
_____ days in a row this period,
and _____ days in a row to date.

The **REWARD** I gave myself for meeting all my weekly goals this period was:

_____
(Color in your **4WEEK BUBBLE** at right)

○ NO, I didn't meet all my weekly goals, but here's what I need to change to succeed next month:
_____

**YES,** I met ALL my weekly goals!

---

Set up your Goals and Color Code for the WEEK of___/___/___ thru ___/___/___ Journaling Week # _____

| **DAILY GOALS** (Your choice of sections below) | **WEEKLY GOALS** | **WEEKLY TAB** |
|---|---|---|
| ○ Same as last week | ○ Same as last week | Review your PowerCircles at week's end |

**My daily food goal is:** _____ **calories**

My color for meeting all my daily food goals:
_____ ( )
_____ ( )
_____ ( )
_____ ( )

I'll meet the goal at left at least _____ times per week

Did I meet my weekly goal at left?

**YES,** I met my weekly goal!
(Color it in)

---

**I'll include these healthy foods each day:**

FoodDot Color        Food Group/Item        Amount

(optional Lean Mode Life Day)

I'll meet the goal at left at least
_____ times per week
_____ times per week
_____ times per week

Did I meet my weekly goal at left?

**YES,** I met my weekly goal!
(Color it in)

---

**I'll color in a** _____ **- free day**
(e.g. sugar-free, pastry-free, soda-free, etc.)

in this color in this spot in my PowerCircles:

I'll meet the goal at left at least _____ times per week

Did I meet my weekly goal at left?

**YES,** I met my weekly goal!
(Color it in)

---

**My daily exercise goal is:** _____

My color for meeting my daily exercise goal is:

I'll meet the goal at left at least _____ times per week

Did I meet my weekly goal at left?

**YES,** I met my weekly goal!
(Color it in)

---

My **4WEEK BUBBLE REWARD** for meeting all my weekly goals will be: _____

# Lean Mode Food Diary **Daily Page** FOR _____ / _____ / _____

| What I ate/drank | Where/When | Quantity | Calories | Fat Grams | Carbs Grams | Fiber Grams | Protein Grams | |
|---|---|---|---|---|---|---|---|---|
| | | | | | | | | |
| | | | | | | | | |
| | | | | | | | | |
| | | | | | | | | |
| | | | | | | | | |
| | | | | | | | | |
| | | | | | | | | |
| | | | | | | | | |
| | | | | | | | | |
| | | | | | | | | |
| | | | | | | | | |
| | | | | | | | | |
| | | | | | | | | |
| **FOOD TOTALS:** | | | | | | | | |

**Color in** the FoodDots above that show healthy eating.
Try to connect-the-FoodDots with color.

| | Where | When | Duration | Distance | | |
|---|---|---|---|---|---|---|
| Exercise | | | | | | |
| **EXERCISE TOTALS:** | | | | | | |

## Color in
## today's PowerCircles!

Met exercise goal today  _____

Days in a row of
Lean Mode journaling  _____

lbs.

Met food goal today  _____

- free day

Glasses of water

# Lean Mode Food Diary **Daily Page**  FOR _____ / _____ / _____

| | What I ate/drank | Where/When | Quantity | Calories | Fat Grams | Carbs Grams | Fiber Grams | Protein Grams | |
|---|---|---|---|---|---|---|---|---|---|
| | | | | | | | | | |
| | | | | | | | | | |
| | | | | | | | | | |
| | | | | | | | | | |
| | | | | | | | | | |
| | | | | | | | | | |
| | | | | | | | | | |
| | | | | | | | | | |
| | | | | | | | | | |
| | | | | | | | | | |
| | | | | | | | | | |
| | | | | | | | | | |
| | | | | | | | | | |
| | | | | | | | | | |
| | | | | | | | | | |

**FOOD TOTALS:**

**Color in** the FoodDots above that show healthy eating.
Try to connect-the-FoodDots with color.

| | Where | When | Duration | Distance |
|---|---|---|---|---|
| Exercise | | | | |

**EXERCISE TOTALS:**

## Color in today's PowerCircles!

Met exercise goal today _____

Days in a row of Lean Mode journaling _____

lbs.

Met food goal today _____

- free day _____

Glasses of water _____

Su   M   Tu   W   Th   F   Sa   Select Day of Week

# Lean Mode Food Diary **Daily Page** FOR _____/_____/_____

| What I ate/drank | Where/When | Quantity | Calories | Fat Grams | Carbs Grams | Fiber Grams | Protein Grams | |
|---|---|---|---|---|---|---|---|---|
| | | | | | | | | |
| | | | | | | | | |
| | | | | | | | | |
| | | | | | | | | |
| | | | | | | | | |
| | | | | | | | | |
| | | | | | | | | |
| | | | | | | | | |
| | | | | | | | | |
| | | | | | | | | |
| | | | | | | | | |
| | | | | | | | | |
| **FOOD TOTALS:** | | | | | | | | |

**Color in** the FoodDots above that show healthy eating.
Try to connect-the-FoodDots with color.

| | Where | When | Duration | Distance | |
|---|---|---|---|---|---|
| Exercise | | | | | |
| **EXERCISE TOTALS:** | | | | | |

# Color in
## today's PowerCircles!

Met exercise goal today _____

Days in a row of
Lean Mode journaling _____    lbs.

Met food goal today _____

- free day _____

Glasses of water _____

Su M Tu W Th F Sa  **Select Day of Week**

# Lean Mode Food Diary **Daily Page** FOR _____ / _____ / _____

| What I ate/drank | Where/When | Quantity | Calories | Fat Grams | Carbs Grams | Fiber Grams | Protein Grams | |
|---|---|---|---|---|---|---|---|---|
| | | | | | | | | |
| | | | | | | | | |
| | | | | | | | | |
| | | | | | | | | |
| | | | | | | | | |
| | | | | | | | | |
| | | | | | | | | |
| | | | | | | | | |
| | | | | | | | | |
| | | | | | | | | |
| | | | | | | | | |
| | | | | | | | | |
| | | | | | | | | |
| | | | | | | | | |
| | | | | | | | | |
| | | **FOOD TOTALS:** | | | | | | |

**Color in** the FoodDots above that show healthy eating.
Try to connect-the-FoodDots with color.

| | Where | When | Duration | Distance | |
|---|---|---|---|---|---|
| Exercise | | | | | |
| | | **EXERCISE TOTALS:** | | | |

## Color in today's PowerCircles!

Met exercise goal today _____

Days in a row of Lean Mode journaling _____

_____ lbs.

Met food goal today _____

- free day _____

Glasses of water _____

# Lean Mode Food Diary **Daily Page** FOR ___ / ___ / ___

| What I ate/drank | Where/When | Quantity | Calories | Fat Grams | Carbs Grams | Fiber Grams | Protein Grams | |
|---|---|---|---|---|---|---|---|---|
| | | | | | | | | |
| | | | | | | | | |
| | | | | | | | | |
| | | | | | | | | |
| | | | | | | | | |
| | | | | | | | | |
| | | | | | | | | |
| | | | | | | | | |
| | | | | | | | | |
| | | | | | | | | |
| | | | | | | | | |
| | | | | | | | | |
| **FOOD TOTALS:** | | | | | | | | |

**Color in** the FoodDots above that show healthy eating.
Try to connect-the-FoodDots with color.

| | Where | When | Duration | Distance | | |
|---|---|---|---|---|---|---|
| Exercise | | | | | | |
| **EXERCISE TOTALS:** | | | | | | |

# Color in
## today's PowerCircles!

Met exercise goal today ___

Met food goal today ___

Days in a row of Lean Mode journaling ___

lbs.

- free day ___

Glasses of water ___

# Lean Mode Food Diary **Daily Page** FOR _____ / _____ / _____

| What I ate/drank | Where/When | Quantity | Calories | Fat Grams | Carbs Grams | Fiber Grams | Protein Grams | |
|---|---|---|---|---|---|---|---|---|
| | | | | | | | | |

**FOOD TOTALS:**

**Color in** the FoodDots above that show healthy eating.
Try to connect-the-FoodDots with color.

| | Where | When | Duration | Distance | |
|---|---|---|---|---|---|
| Exercise | | | | | |

**EXERCISE TOTALS:**

# Color in
## today's PowerCircles!

Met exercise goal today

Days in a row of
Lean Mode journaling

lbs.

Met food goal today

- free day

Glasses of water

Su M Tu W Th F Sa  Select Day of Week

# Lean Mode Food Diary **Daily Page** FOR _____ / ___ / _____

| | What I ate/drank | Where/When | Quantity | Calories | Fat Grams | Carbs Grams | Fiber Grams | Protein Grams | |
|---|---|---|---|---|---|---|---|---|---|
| | | | | | | | | | |
| | | | | | | | | | |
| | | | | | | | | | |
| | | | | | | | | | |
| | | | | | | | | | |
| | | | | | | | | | |
| | | | | | | | | | |
| | | | | | | | | | |
| | | | | | | | | | |
| | | | | | | | | | |
| | | | | | | | | | |
| | | | | | | | | | |
| | | | | | | | | | |
| | **FOOD TOTALS:** | | | | | | | | |

**Color in** the FoodDots above that show healthy eating.
Try to connect-the-FoodDots with color.

| | Where | When | Duration | Distance |
|---|---|---|---|---|
| Exercise | | | | |
| **EXERCISE TOTALS:** | | | | |

## Color in today's PowerCircles!

Met exercise goal today _____

Met food goal today _____

- free day _____

Days in a row of Lean Mode journaling _____

lbs.

Glasses of water _____

# Fill in Your **Color Code & Goals Page**

Take baby steps! Gradually build better habits by setting realistic goals here.

**NOTES:**

Set up your Goals and Color Code for the WEEK of ____/____/____ thru ____/____/____ Journaling Week # _____

| **DAILY GOALS** (Your choice of sections below)<br>◯ Same as last week | **WEEKLY GOALS**<br>◯ Same as last week | **WEEKLY TAB**<br>Review your PowerCircles<br>at week's end |
|---|---|---|
| **My daily food goal is:** _____ **calories**<br><br>My color for meeting all<br>my daily food goals:<br>_____ (    )<br>_____ (    )<br>_____ (    )<br>_____ (    ) | I'll meet the goal at left<br>at least _____ times<br>per week | Did I<br>meet<br>my<br>weekly<br>goal<br>at left?   **YES,** I met my weekly goal!<br>(Color it in) |
| **I'll include these healthy foods each day:**<br>FoodDot Color    Food Group/Item    Amount<br><br><br>Optional Lean Mode Lite Day | I'll meet the goal at left<br>at least<br><br>_____ times per week<br>_____ times per week<br>_____ times per week | Did I<br>meet<br>my<br>weekly<br>goal<br>at left?   **YES,** I met my weekly goal!<br>(Color it in) |
| **I'll color in a** _____ **- free day**<br>(e.g. sugar-free, pastry-free, soda-free, etc.)<br>in this color in this spot in<br>my PowerCircles: | I'll meet the goal at left<br>at least _____ times<br>per week | Did I<br>meet<br>my<br>weekly<br>goal<br>at left?   **YES,** I met my weekly goal!<br>(Color it in) |
| **My daily exercise goal is:** _____<br>_____<br><br>My color for meeting my<br>daily exercise goal is: | I'll meet the goal at left<br>at least _____ times<br>per week | Did I<br>meet<br>my<br>weekly<br>goal<br>at left?   **YES,** I met my weekly goal!<br>(Color it in) |

My **4WEEK BUBBLE REWARD** for meeting all my weekly goals will be: _____

# Lean Mode Food Diary **Daily Page** FOR ____ / ____ / ____

| What I ate/drank | Where/When | Quantity | Calories | Fat Grams | Carbs Grams | Fiber Grams | Protein Grams |
|---|---|---|---|---|---|---|---|
| | | | | | | | |
| | | | | | | | |
| | | | | | | | |
| | | | | | | | |
| | | | | | | | |
| | | | | | | | |
| | | | | | | | |
| | | | | | | | |
| | | | | | | | |
| | | | | | | | |
| | | | | | | | |
| | | | | | | | |
| **FOOD TOTALS:** | | | | | | | |

**Color in** the FoodDots above that show healthy eating. Try to connect-the-FoodDots with color.

| | Where | When | Duration | Distance |
|---|---|---|---|---|
| Exercise | | | | |
| **EXERCISE TOTALS:** | | | | |

## Color in today's PowerCircles!

Met exercise goal today ____

Days in a row of Lean Mode journaling ____   ____ lbs.

Met food goal today ____

- free day ____

Glasses of water ____

Su M Tu W Th F Sa  **Select Day of Week**

# Lean Mode Food Diary **Daily Page** FOR _____ / _____ / _____

| | What I ate/drank | Where/When | Quantity | Calories | Fat Grams | Carbs Grams | Fiber Grams | Protein Grams | |
|---|---|---|---|---|---|---|---|---|---|
| | | | | | | | | | |
| | | | | | | | | | |
| | | | | | | | | | |
| | | | | | | | | | |
| | | | | | | | | | |
| | | | | | | | | | |
| | | | | | | | | | |
| | | | | | | | | | |
| | | | | | | | | | |
| | | | | | | | | | |
| | | | | | | | | | |
| | | | | | | | | | |
| | | | | | | | | | |
| | | | | | | | | | |
| | **FOOD TOTALS:** | | | | | | | | |

**Color in** the FoodDots above that show healthy eating.
Try to connect-the-FoodDots with color.

| | Where | When | Duration | Distance |
|---|---|---|---|---|
| Exercise | | | | |
| | | | | |
| **EXERCISE TOTALS:** | | | | |

## Color in today's PowerCircles!

Met exercise goal today _____

Days in a row of Lean Mode journaling _____

_____ lbs.

Met food goal today _____

- free day _____

Glasses of water _____

# Lean Mode Food Diary **Daily Page** FOR ____ / ____ / ____

| What I ate/drank | Where/When | Quantity | Calories | Fat Grams | Carbs Grams | Fiber Grams | Protein Grams |
|---|---|---|---|---|---|---|---|
| | | | | | | | |
| | | | | | | | |
| | | | | | | | |
| | | | | | | | |
| | | | | | | | |
| | | | | | | | |
| | | | | | | | |
| | | | | | | | |
| | | | | | | | |
| | | | | | | | |
| | | | | | | | |
| | | | | | | | |
| | | | | | | | |
| **FOOD TOTALS:** | | | | | | | |

**Color in** the FoodDots above that show healthy eating.
Try to connect-the-FoodDots with color.

| Exercise | Where | When | Duration | Distance | | |
|---|---|---|---|---|---|---|
| | | | | | | |
| **EXERCISE TOTALS:** | | | | | | |

## Color in today's PowerCircles!

Met exercise goal today _____

Days in a row of Lean Mode journaling _____

_____ lbs.

Met food goal today _____

_____ - free day

Glasses of water _____

Su  M  Tu  W  Th  F  Sa   Select Day
of Week

# Lean Mode Food Diary **Daily Page** FOR _____ / _____ / _____

| What I ate/drank | Where/When | Quantity | Calories | Fat Grams | Carbs Grams | Fiber Grams | Protein Grams | |
|---|---|---|---|---|---|---|---|---|
| | | | | | | | | |
| | | | | | | | | |
| | | | | | | | | |
| | | | | | | | | |
| | | | | | | | | |
| | | | | | | | | |
| | | | | | | | | |
| | | | | | | | | |
| | | | | | | | | |
| | | | | | | | | |
| **FOOD TOTALS:** | | | | | | | | |

**Color in** the FoodDots above that show healthy eating.
Try to connect-the-FoodDots with color.

| | Where | When | Duration | Distance |
|---|---|---|---|---|
| Exercise | | | | |
| **EXERCISE TOTALS:** | | | | |

# Color in
## today's PowerCircles!

Met exercise goal today _____

Days in a row of
Lean Mode journaling _____

lbs.

Met food goal today _____

- free day _____

Glasses of water _____

Su  M  Tu  W  Th  F  Sa   Select Day of Week

# Lean Mode Food Diary **Daily Page** FOR _____ / _____ / _____

| | What I ate/drank | Where/When | Quantity | Calories | Fat Grams | Carbs Grams | Fiber Grams | Protein Grams | |
|---|---|---|---|---|---|---|---|---|---|
| | | | | | | | | | |
| | | | | | | | | | |
| | | | | | | | | | |
| | | | | | | | | | |
| | | | | | | | | | |
| | | | | | | | | | |
| | | | | | | | | | |
| | | | | | | | | | |
| | | | | | | | | | |
| | | | | | | | | | |
| | | | | | | | | | |
| | | | | | | | | | |
| | | | | | | | | | |
| | **FOOD TOTALS:** | | | | | | | | |

**Color in** the FoodDots above that show healthy eating.
Try to connect-the-FoodDots with color.

| | Where | When | Duration | Distance | |
|---|---|---|---|---|---|
| Exercise | | | | | |
| **EXERCISE TOTALS:** | | | | | |

# Color in
## today's PowerCircles!

Met exercise goal today _____

Days in a row of
Lean Mode journaling _____

lbs.

Met food goal today _____

- free day _____

Glasses of water _____

Su  M  Tu  W  Th  F  Sa   Select Day
                           of Week

# Lean Mode Food Diary **Daily Page** FOR _____ / _____ / _____

| What I ate/drank | Where/When | Quantity | Calories | Fat Grams | Carbs Grams | Fiber Grams | Protein Grams |
|---|---|---|---|---|---|---|---|
|  |  |  |  |  |  |  |  |
|  |  |  |  |  |  |  |  |
|  |  |  |  |  |  |  |  |
|  |  |  |  |  |  |  |  |
|  |  |  |  |  |  |  |  |
|  |  |  |  |  |  |  |  |
|  |  |  |  |  |  |  |  |
|  |  |  |  |  |  |  |  |
|  |  |  |  |  |  |  |  |
| **FOOD TOTALS:** |  |  |  |  |  |  |  |

**Color in** the FoodDots above that show healthy eating.
Try to connect-the-FoodDots with color.

| | Where | When | Duration | Distance |
|---|---|---|---|---|
| Exercise |  |  |  |  |
| **EXERCISE TOTALS:** |  |  |  |  |

## Color in today's PowerCircles!

Met exercise goal today _____

Days in a row of
Lean Mode journaling _____          lbs.

Met food goal today _____

- free day _____

Glasses of water _____

Su M Tu W Th F Sa    Select Day of Week

# Lean Mode Food Diary **Daily Page**   FOR _____ / _____ / _____

| What I ate/drank | Where/When | Quantity | Calories | Fat Grams | Carbs Grams | Fiber Grams | Protein Grams | |
|---|---|---|---|---|---|---|---|---|
| | | | | | | | | |
| | | | | | | | | |
| | | | | | | | | |
| | | | | | | | | |
| | | | | | | | | |
| | | | | | | | | |
| | | | | | | | | |
| | | | | | | | | |
| | | | | | | | | |
| | | | | | | | | |
| | | | | | | | | |
| | | | | | | | | |
| | | | | | | | | |
| **FOOD TOTALS:** | | | | | | | | |

**Color in** the FoodDots above that show healthy eating.
Try to connect-the-FoodDots with color.

| | Where | When | Duration | Distance | | |
|---|---|---|---|---|---|---|
| Exercise | | | | | | |
| **EXERCISE TOTALS:** | | | | | | |

## Color in today's PowerCircles!

Met exercise goal today _____

Met food goal today _____

- free day _____

Days in a row of Lean Mode journaling _____

_____ lbs.

Glasses of water _____

# Fill in Your **Color Code & Goals Page**

Take baby steps! Gradually build better habits by setting realistic goals here.

**NOTES:**

Set up your Goals and Color Code for the WEEK of ___/___/___ thru ___/___/___    Journaling Week # _____

| **DAILY GOALS** (Your choice of sections below)<br>○ Same as last week | **WEEKLY GOALS**<br>○ Same as last week | **WEEKLY TAB**<br>Review your PowerCircles at week's end |
|---|---|---|
| **My daily food goal is:** _____ **calories**<br><br>My color for meeting all<br>my daily food goals:<br>( )  ( )  ( )  ( )  ( ) | I'll meet the goal at left<br>at least _____ times<br>per week | Did I meet my weekly goal at left?<br>**YES,** I met my weekly goal!<br>(Color it in) |
| **I'll include these healthy foods each day:**<br>FoodDot Color    Food Group/Item    Amount<br><br>Optional Lean Mode Lite Day | I'll meet the goal at left<br>at least<br>_____ times per week<br>_____ times per week<br>_____ times per week | Did I meet my weekly goal at left?<br>**YES,** I met my weekly goal!<br>(Color it in) |
| **I'll color in a** _____ **- free day**<br>(e.g. sugar-free, pastry-free, soda-free, etc.)<br>in this color in this spot in<br>my PowerCircles: | I'll meet the goal at left<br>at least _____ times<br>per week | Did I meet my weekly goal at left?<br>**YES,** I met my weekly goal!<br>(Color it in) |
| **My daily exercise goal is:** _____<br><br>My color for meeting my<br>daily exercise goal is: | I'll meet the goal at left<br>at least _____ times<br>per week | Did I meet my weekly goal at left?<br>**YES,** I met my weekly goal!<br>(Color it in) |

My **4WEEK BUBBLE REWARD** for meeting all my weekly goals will be: _____

# Lean Mode Food Diary **Daily Page** FOR _____ / _____ / _____

| | What I ate/drank | Where/When | Quantity | Calories | Fat Grams | Carbs Grams | Fiber Grams | Protein Grams | |
|---|---|---|---|---|---|---|---|---|---|
| | | | | | | | | | |
| | | | | | | | | | |
| | | | | | | | | | |
| | | | | | | | | | |
| | | | | | | | | | |
| | | | | | | | | | |
| | | | | | | | | | |
| | | | | | | | | | |
| | | | | | | | | | |
| | | | | | | | | | |
| | | | | | | | | | |
| | | | | | | | | | |
| | | | | | | | | | |
| | | | | | | | | | |
| | **FOOD TOTALS:** | | | | | | | | |

**Color in** the FoodDots above that show healthy eating.
Try to connect-the-FoodDots with color.

| | Where | When | Duration | Distance | | |
|---|---|---|---|---|---|---|
| Exercise | | | | | | |
| **EXERCISE TOTALS:** | | | | | | |

# Color in
## today's PowerCircles!

Met exercise goal today _____

Days in a row of
Lean Mode journaling _____

lbs.

Met food goal today _____

- free day _____

Glasses of water _____

Su  M  Tu  W  Th  F  Sa    Select Day
of Week

# Lean Mode Food Diary **Daily Page**  FOR ____ / ____ / ____

| What I ate/drank | Where/When | Quantity | Calories | Fat Grams | Carbs Grams | Fiber Grams | Protein Grams | |
|---|---|---|---|---|---|---|---|---|
| | | | | | | | | |
| | | | | | | | | |
| | | | | | | | | |
| | | | | | | | | |
| | | | | | | | | |
| | | | | | | | | |
| | | | | | | | | |
| | | | | | | | | |
| | | | | | | | | |
| | | | | | | | | |
| | | | | | | | | |
| | | | | | | | | |
| | | | | | | | | |
| | | | | | | | | |
| | | | | | | | | |
| | | | | | | | | |
| **FOOD TOTALS:** | | | | | | | | |

**Color in** the FoodDots above that show healthy eating.
Try to connect-the-FoodDots with color.

| | Where | When | Duration | Distance |
|---|---|---|---|---|
| Exercise | | | | |
| **EXERCISE TOTALS:** | | | | |

## Color in
today's PowerCircles!

Met exercise goal today _____

Days in a row of
Lean Mode journaling _____

_____ lbs.

Met food goal today _____

- free day _____

Glasses of water _____

# Lean Mode Food Diary **Daily Page** FOR ____ / ____ / ____

| What I ate/drank | Where/When | Quantity | Calories | Fat Grams | Carbs Grams | Fiber Grams | Protein Grams |
|---|---|---|---|---|---|---|---|
| | | | | | | | |
| | | | | | | | |
| | | | | | | | |
| | | | | | | | |
| | | | | | | | |
| | | | | | | | |
| | | | | | | | |
| | | | | | | | |
| | | | | | | | |
| | | | | | | | |
| | | | | | | | |
| | | | | | | | |
| | | | | | | | |
| | | | | | | | |
| | | | | | | | |
| **FOOD TOTALS:** | | | | | | | |

**Color in** the FoodDots above that show healthy eating.
Try to connect-the-FoodDots with color.

| | Where | When | Duration | Distance | |
|---|---|---|---|---|---|
| Exercise | | | | | |
| **EXERCISE TOTALS:** | | | | | |

## Color in
today's PowerCircles!

Met exercise goal today _____

Met food goal today _____

- free day

Days in a row of
Lean Mode journaling _____

lbs.

Glasses of water

Su  M  Tu  W  Th  F  Sa    Select Day
of Week

# Lean Mode Food Diary **Daily Page**  FOR  _____ / _____ / _____

| What I ate/drank | Where/When | Quantity | Calories | Fat Grams | Carbs Grams | Fiber Grams | Protein Grams | |
|---|---|---|---|---|---|---|---|---|
| | | | | | | | | |
| | | | | | | | | |
| | | | | | | | | |
| | | | | | | | | |
| | | | | | | | | |
| | | | | | | | | |
| | | | | | | | | |
| | | | | | | | | |
| | | | | | | | | |
| | | | | | | | | |
| | | | | | | | | |
| | | | | | | | | |

**FOOD TOTALS:**

**Color in** the FoodDots above that show healthy eating.
Try to connect-the-FoodDots with color.

| | Where | When | Duration | Distance | |
|---|---|---|---|---|---|
| Exercise | | | | | |

**EXERCISE TOTALS:**

# Color in
## today's PowerCircles!

Met exercise goal today _____

Days in a row of
Lean Mode journaling _____

lbs.

Met food goal today _____

- free day _____

Glasses of water _____

# Lean Mode Food Diary **Daily Page** FOR _____ / _____ / _____

| | What I ate/drank | Where/When | Quantity | Calories | Fat Grams | Carbs Grams | Fiber Grams | Protein Grams | |
|---|---|---|---|---|---|---|---|---|---|
| | | | | | | | | | |
| | | | | | | | | | |
| | | | | | | | | | |
| | | | | | | | | | |
| | | | | | | | | | |
| | | | | | | | | | |
| | | | | | | | | | |
| | | | | | | | | | |
| | | | | | | | | | |
| | | | | | | | | | |
| | | | | | | | | | |
| | | | | | | | | | |
| | | | | | | | | | |
| | **FOOD TOTALS:** | | | | | | | | |

**Color in** the FoodDots above that show healthy eating.
Try to connect-the-FoodDots with color.

| | Where | When | Duration | Distance | |
|---|---|---|---|---|---|
| Exercise | | | | | |
| **EXERCISE TOTALS:** | | | | | |

# Color in
## today's PowerCircles!

Met exercise goal today _____

Days in a row of
Lean Mode journaling _____

lbs.

Met food goal today _____

- free day _____

Glasses of water _____

Su  M  Tu  W  Th  F  Sa    Select Day
of Week

# Lean Mode Food Diary **Daily Page**  FOR  _____ / _____ / _____

| | What I ate/drank | Where/When | Quantity | Calories | Fat Grams | Carbs Grams | Fiber Grams | Protein Grams | |
|---|---|---|---|---|---|---|---|---|---|
| | | | | | | | | | |
| | | | | | | | | | |
| | | | | | | | | | |
| | | | | | | | | | |
| | | | | | | | | | |
| | | | | | | | | | |
| | | | | | | | | | |
| | | | | | | | | | |
| | | | | | | | | | |
| | | | | | | | | | |
| | | | | | | | | | |
| | **FOOD TOTALS:** | | | | | | | | |

**Color in** the FoodDots above that show healthy eating.
Try to connect-the-FoodDots with color.

| | Where | When | Duration | Distance | |
|---|---|---|---|---|---|
| Exercise | | | | | |
| **EXERCISE TOTALS:** | | | | | |

# Color in
## today's PowerCircles!

Met exercise goal today _____

Days in a row of
Lean Mode journaling _____        lbs.

Met food goal today _____

- free day _____

Glasses of water _____

# Lean Mode Food Diary **Daily Page**  FOR _____ / _____ / _____

| What I ate/drank | Where/When | Quantity | Calories | Fat Grams | Carbs Grams | Fiber Grams | Protein Grams | |
|---|---|---|---|---|---|---|---|---|
| | | | | | | | | |
| | | | | | | | | |
| | | | | | | | | |
| | | | | | | | | |
| | | | | | | | | |
| | | | | | | | | |
| | | | | | | | | |
| | | | | | | | | |
| | | | | | | | | |
| | | | | | | | | |
| | | | | | | | | |
| | | | | | | | | |
| | | | | | | | | |
| | | | | | | | | |
| | | | | | | | | |
| **FOOD TOTALS:** | | | | | | | | |

**Color in** the FoodDots above that show healthy eating.
Try to connect-the-FoodDots with color.

| | Where | When | Duration | Distance | |
|---|---|---|---|---|---|
| Exercise | | | | | |
| | | | | | |
| **EXERCISE TOTALS:** | | | | | |

## Color in today's PowerCircles!

Met exercise goal today _____

Days in a row of Lean Mode journaling _____

_____ lbs.

Met food goal today _____

- free day _____

Glasses of water _____

# Fill in Your **Color Code & Goals Page**

Take baby steps! Gradually build better habits by setting realistic goals here.

**NOTES:**

Set up your Goals and Color Code for the WEEK of _ _ _ _ / _ _ _ / _ _ _ _ thru _ _ _ _ / _ _ _ / _ _ _ _   Journaling Week # _ _ _ _ _ _

| **DAILY GOALS** (Your choice of sections below) ○ Same as last week | **WEEKLY GOALS** ○ Same as last week | **WEEKLY TAB** Review your PowerCircles at week's end |
|---|---|---|
| **My daily food goal is:** _____ calories My color for meeting all my daily food goals: ( ) ( ) ( ) ( ) | I'll meet the goal at left at least _____ times per week | Did I meet my weekly goal at left? **YES,** I met my weekly goal! (Color it in) |
| **I'll include these healthy foods each day:** FoodDot Color   Food Group/Item   Amount _Optional Lean Mode Lite Day_ | I'll meet the goal at left at least _____ times per week _____ times per week _____ times per week | Did I meet my weekly goal at left? **YES,** I met my weekly goal! (Color it in) |
| **I'll color in a** _____ **- free day** (e.g. sugar-free, pastry-free, soda-free, etc.) in this color in this spot in my PowerCircles: | I'll meet the goal at left at least _____ times per week | Did I meet my weekly goal at left? **YES,** I met my weekly goal! (Color it in) |
| **My daily exercise goal is:** _____ My color for meeting my daily exercise goal is: | I'll meet the goal at left at least _____ times per week | Did I meet my weekly goal at left? **YES,** I met my weekly goal! (Color it in) |

My **4WEEK BUBBLE REWARD** for meeting all my weekly goals will be: _____

Su  M  Tu  W  Th  F  Sa   Select Day of Week

# Lean Mode Food Diary **Daily Page** FOR _____ / _____ / _____

| | What I ate/drank | Where/When | Quantity | Calories | Fat Grams | Carbs Grams | Fiber Grams | Protein Grams | |
|---|---|---|---|---|---|---|---|---|---|
| | | | | | | | | | |
| | | | | | | | | | |
| | | | | | | | | | |
| | | | | | | | | | |
| | | | | | | | | | |
| | | | | | | | | | |
| | | | | | | | | | |
| | | | | | | | | | |
| | | | | | | | | | |
| | | | | | | | | | |
| | | | | | | | | | |
| | | | | | | | | | |
| | | | | | | | | | |
| | | | | | | | | | |
| | **FOOD TOTALS:** | | | | | | | | |

**Color in** the FoodDots above that show healthy eating.
Try to connect-the-FoodDots with color.

| | Where | When | Duration | Distance | |
|---|---|---|---|---|---|
| Exercise | | | | | |
| | **EXERCISE TOTALS:** | | | | |

# Color in
## today's PowerCircles!

Met exercise goal today _____

Days in a row of
Lean Mode journaling _____

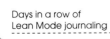

lbs.

Met food goal today _____

- free day _____

Glasses of water _____

Su  M  Tu  W  Th  F  Sa   Select Day
of Week

# Lean Mode Food Diary **Daily Page** FOR ___ / ___ / ___

| What I ate/drank | Where/When | Quantity | Calories | Fat Grams | Carbs Grams | Fiber Grams | Protein Grams | |
|---|---|---|---|---|---|---|---|---|
| | | | | | | | | |
| | | | | | | | | |
| | | | | | | | | |
| | | | | | | | | |
| | | | | | | | | |
| | | | | | | | | |
| | | | | | | | | |
| | | | | | | | | |
| | | | | | | | | |
| | | | | | | | | |
| | | | | | | | | |
| | | | | | | | | |
| | | | | | | | | |
| | | | | | | | | |
| **FOOD TOTALS:** | | | | | | | | |

**Color in** the FoodDots above that show healthy eating.
Try to connect-the-FoodDots with color.

| | Where | When | Duration | Distance | |
|---|---|---|---|---|---|
| Exercise | | | | | |
| **EXERCISE TOTALS:** | | | | | |

# Color in
## today's PowerCircles!

Met exercise goal today ___

Days in a row of
Lean Mode journaling ___          ___ lbs.

Met food goal today ___

- free day ___

Glasses of water ___

# Lean Mode Food Diary **Daily Page** FOR _____/_____/_____

| What I ate/drank | Where/When | Quantity | Calories | Fat Grams | Carbs Grams | Fiber Grams | Protein Grams | |
|---|---|---|---|---|---|---|---|---|
| | | | | | | | | |
| | | | | | | | | |
| | | | | | | | | |
| | | | | | | | | |
| | | | | | | | | |
| | | | | | | | | |
| | | | | | | | | |
| | | | | | | | | |
| | | | | | | | | |
| | | | | | | | | |
| | | | | | | | | |
| | | | | | | | | |
| | | | | | | | | |
| **FOOD TOTALS:** | | | | | | | | |

**Color in** the FoodDots above that show healthy eating.
Try to connect-the-FoodDots with color.

| | Where | When | Duration | Distance | | | |
|---|---|---|---|---|---|---|---|
| Exercise | | | | | | | |
| | | | | | | | |
| **EXERCISE TOTALS:** | | | | | | | |

# Color in
## today's PowerCircles!

Met exercise goal today _____

Met food goal today _____

- free day _____

Days in a row of
Lean Mode journaling _____    lbs.

Glasses of water _____

Su  M  Tu  W  Th  F  Sa  **Select Day of Week**

# Lean Mode Food Diary **Daily Page** FOR _____ / _____ / _____

| What I ate/drank | Where/When | Quantity | Calories | Fat Grams | Carbs Grams | Fiber Grams | Protein Grams |
|---|---|---|---|---|---|---|---|
| | | | | | | | |
| | | | | | | | |
| | | | | | | | |
| | | | | | | | |
| | | | | | | | |
| | | | | | | | |
| | | | | | | | |
| | | | | | | | |
| | | | | | | | |
| **FOOD TOTALS:** | | | | | | | |

**Color in** the FoodDots above that show healthy eating.
Try to connect-the-FoodDots with color.

| | Where | When | Duration | Distance |
|---|---|---|---|---|
| Exercise | | | | |
| **EXERCISE TOTALS:** | | | | |

## Color in
today's PowerCircles!

Met exercise goal today _____

Days in a row of
Lean Mode journaling _____          lbs.

Met food goal today _____

_____ - free day

Glasses of water _____

Su M Tu W Th F Sa Select Day of Week

# Lean Mode Food Diary **Daily Page** FOR _____ / _____ / _____

| What I ate/drank | Where/When | Quantity | Calories | Fat Grams | Carbs Grams | Fiber Grams | Protein Grams | |
|---|---|---|---|---|---|---|---|---|
| | | | | | | | | |
| | | | | | | | | |
| | | | | | | | | |
| | | | | | | | | |
| | | | | | | | | |
| | | | | | | | | |
| | | | | | | | | |
| | | | | | | | | |
| | | | | | | | | |
| | | | | | | | | |
| | | | | | | | | |
| **FOOD TOTALS:** | | | | | | | | |

**Color in** the FoodDots above that show healthy eating.
Try to connect-the-FoodDots with color.

| | Where | When | Duration | Distance | |
|---|---|---|---|---|---|
| Exercise | | | | | |
| **EXERCISE TOTALS:** | | | | | |

## Color in today's PowerCircles!

Met exercise goal today _____

Days in a row of Lean Mode journaling _____

_____ lbs.

Met food goal today _____

_____ - free day

_____ Glasses of water

# Lean Mode Food Diary **Daily Page** FOR ___ / ___ / ___

| What I ate/drank | Where/When | Quantity | Calories | Fat Grams | Carbs Grams | Fiber Grams | Protein Grams |
|---|---|---|---|---|---|---|---|
|  |  |  |  |  |  |  |  |
|  |  |  |  |  |  |  |  |
|  |  |  |  |  |  |  |  |
|  |  |  |  |  |  |  |  |
|  |  |  |  |  |  |  |  |
|  |  |  |  |  |  |  |  |
|  |  |  |  |  |  |  |  |
|  |  |  |  |  |  |  |  |
|  |  |  |  |  |  |  |  |
|  |  |  |  |  |  |  |  |
|  |  |  |  |  |  |  |  |
| **FOOD TOTALS:** |  |  |  |  |  |  |  |

**Color in** the FoodDots above that show healthy eating.
Try to connect-the-FoodDots with color.

| | Where | When | Duration | Distance |
|---|---|---|---|---|
| Exercise |  |  |  |  |
| **EXERCISE TOTALS:** |  |  |  |  |

# Color in
## today's PowerCircles!

Met exercise goal today _____

Met food goal today _____

Days in a row of
Lean Mode journaling _____

lbs.

- free day _____

Glasses of water _____

Su M Tu W Th F Sa   Select Day of Week

# Lean Mode Food Diary **Daily Page** FOR _____ / _____ / _____

| What I ate/drank | Where/When | Quantity | Calories | Fat Grams | Carbs Grams | Fiber Grams | Protein Grams |
|---|---|---|---|---|---|---|---|
| | | | | | | | |
| | | | | | | | |
| | | | | | | | |
| | | | | | | | |
| | | | | | | | |
| | | | | | | | |
| | | | | | | | |
| | | | | | | | |
| | | | | | | | |
| | | | | | | | |
| | | | | | | | |
| | | | | | | | |
| | | | | | | | |
| | | | | | | | |
| **FOOD TOTALS:** | | | | | | | |

**Color in** the FoodDots above that show healthy eating.
Try to connect-the-FoodDots with color.

| | Where | When | Duration | Distance | |
|---|---|---|---|---|---|
| Exercise | | | | | |
| **EXERCISE TOTALS:** | | | | | |

## Color in
today's PowerCircles!

Met exercise goal today _____

Met food goal today _____

- free day _____

Days in a row of
Lean Mode journaling _____   lbs.

Glasses of water _____

# Complete Your **4Week Bubble**

Look back over your Weekly Tabs for the past 4 weeks and tally the results.

**4WEEK BUBBLE RECAP:** ___/___/___ thru ___/___/___

|  | Start | End | + or − |
|---|---|---|---|
| Weight | | | |
| | | | |
| | | | |

**Yay!** I journaled every day

I journaled _____ days this period, _____ days in a row this period, and _____ days in a row to date.

The **REWARD** I gave myself for meeting all my weekly goals this period was:

_____
(Color in your **4WEEK BUBBLE** at right)

**YES,** I met ALL my weekly goals!

O NO, I didn't meet all my weekly goals, but here's what I need to change to succeed next month:

_____

Set up your Goals and Color Code for the WEEK of ___/___/___ thru ___/___/___ Journaling Week # _____

| **DAILY GOALS** (Your choice of sections below) | **WEEKLY GOALS** | **WEEKLY TAB** |
|---|---|---|
| O Same as last week | O Same as last week | Review your PowerCircles at week's end |
| **My daily food goal is:** _____ **calories** <br><br> My color for meeting all my daily food goals: <br> ( ) <br> ( ) <br> ( ) <br> ( ) | I'll meet the goal at left at least _____ times per week | Did I meet my weekly goal at left? <br> **YES,** I met my weekly goal! <br> (Color it in) |
| **I'll include these healthy foods each day:** <br> FoodDot Color  Food Group/Item  Amount <br><br> Optional Lean Mode Lite Day | I'll meet the goal at left at least <br> _____ times per week <br> _____ times per week <br> _____ times per week | Did I meet my weekly goal at left? <br> **YES,** I met my weekly goal! <br> (Color it in) |
| **I'll color in a** _____ **- free day** <br> (e.g. sugar-free, pastry-free, soda-free, etc.) <br> in this color in this spot in my PowerCircles: | I'll meet the goal at left at least _____ times per week | Did I meet my weekly goal at left? <br> **YES,** I met my weekly goal! <br> (Color it in) |
| **My daily exercise goal is:** _____ <br><br> My color for meeting my daily exercise goal is: | I'll meet the goal at left at least _____ times per week | Did I meet my weekly goal at left? <br> **YES,** I met my weekly goal! <br> (Color it in) |

My **4WEEK BUBBLE REWARD** for meeting all my weekly goals will be: _____

# Lean Mode Food Diary **Daily Page** FOR ___ / ___ / ___

| | What I ate/drank | Where/When | Quantity | Calories | Fat Grams | Carbs Grams | Fiber Grams | Protein Grams | |
|---|---|---|---|---|---|---|---|---|---|
| | | | | | | | | | |
| | | | | | | | | | |
| | | | | | | | | | |
| | | | | | | | | | |
| | | | | | | | | | |
| | | | | | | | | | |
| | | | | | | | | | |
| | | | | | | | | | |
| | | | | | | | | | |
| | | | | | | | | | |
| | **FOOD TOTALS:** | | | | | | | | |

**Color in** the FoodDots above that show healthy eating. Try to connect-the-FoodDots with color.

| | Where | When | Duration | Distance | | |
|---|---|---|---|---|---|---|
| Exercise | | | | | | |
| **EXERCISE TOTALS:** | | | | | | |

# Color in
## today's PowerCircles!

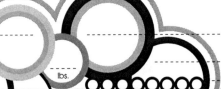

Met exercise goal today ____

Days in a row of
Lean Mode journaling ____

____ lbs.

Met food goal today ____

- free day ____

Glasses of water ____

Su M Tu W Th F Sa  Select Day of Week

# Lean Mode Food Diary **Daily Page** FOR ___ / ___ / ___

| What I ate/drank | Where/When | Quantity | Calories | Fat Grams | Carbs Grams | Fiber Grams | Protein Grams | |
|---|---|---|---|---|---|---|---|---|
| | | | | | | | | |
| | | | | | | | | |
| | | | | | | | | |
| | | | | | | | | |
| | | | | | | | | |
| | | | | | | | | |
| | | | | | | | | |
| | | | | | | | | |
| | | | | | | | | |
| | | | | | | | | |
| | | | | | | | | |
| | | | | | | | | |
| **FOOD TOTALS:** | | | | | | | | |

**Color in** the FoodDots above that show healthy eating.
Try to connect-the-FoodDots with color.

| | Where | When | Duration | Distance | |
|---|---|---|---|---|---|
| Exercise | | | | | |
| | **EXERCISE TOTALS:** | | | | |

## Color in
### today's PowerCircles!

Met exercise goal today ___

Days in a row of
Lean Mode journaling ___        lbs.

Met food goal today ___

- free day ___

Glasses of water ___

# Lean Mode Food Diary **Daily Page** FOR _____ / _____ / _____

| What I ate/drank | Where/When | Quantity | Calories | Fat Grams | Carbs Grams | Fiber Grams | Protein Grams | |
|---|---|---|---|---|---|---|---|---|
| | | | | | | | | |
| | | | | | | | | |
| | | | | | | | | |
| | | | | | | | | |
| | | | | | | | | |
| | | | | | | | | |
| | | | | | | | | |
| | | | | | | | | |
| | | | | | | | | |
| | | | | | | | | |
| | | | | | | | | |
| | | | | | | | | |
| | | | | | | | | |
| | | | | | | | | |
| **FOOD TOTALS:** | | | | | | | | |

**Color in** the FoodDots above that show healthy eating.
Try to connect-the-FoodDots with color.

| | Where | When | Duration | Distance | |
|---|---|---|---|---|---|
| Exercise | | | | | |
| | | | | | |
| **EXERCISE TOTALS:** | | | | | |

# Color in
## today's PowerCircles!

Met exercise goal today _____

Met food goal today _____

- free day _____

Days in a row of
Lean Mode journaling _____    lbs.

Glasses of water _____

Su  M  Tu  W  Th  F  Sa  Select Day
of Week

# Lean Mode Food Diary **Daily Page** FOR _____ / _____ / _____

| What I ate/drank | Where/When | Quantity | Calories | Fat Grams | Carbs Grams | Fiber Grams | Protein Grams |
|---|---|---|---|---|---|---|---|
| | | | | | | | |
| | | | | | | | |
| | | | | | | | |
| | | | | | | | |
| | | | | | | | |
| | | | | | | | |
| | | | | | | | |
| | | | | | | | |
| | | | | | | | |
| | | | | | | | |
| | | | | | | | |
| **FOOD TOTALS:** | | | | | | | |

**Color in** the FoodDots above that show healthy eating.
Try to connect-the-FoodDots with color.

| | Where | When | Duration | Distance |
|---|---|---|---|---|
| Exercise | | | | |
| **EXERCISE TOTALS:** | | | | |

# Color in
## today's PowerCircles!

Met exercise goal today _____

Met food goal today _____

- free day _____

Days in a row of
Lean Mode journaling _____ lbs.

Glasses of water _____

# Lean Mode Food Diary **Daily Page** FOR ___ / ___ / ___

| | What I ate/drank | Where/When | Quantity | Calories | Fat Grams | Carbs Grams | Fiber Grams | Protein Grams | |
|---|---|---|---|---|---|---|---|---|---|
| | | | | | | | | | |
| | | | | | | | | | |
| | **FOOD TOTALS:** | | | | | | | | |

**Color in** the FoodDots above that show healthy eating.
Try to connect-the-FoodDots with color.

| | Where | When | Duration | Distance | |
|---|---|---|---|---|---|
| Exercise | | | | | |
| | **EXERCISE TOTALS:** | | | | |

## Color in today's PowerCircles!

Met exercise goal today _____

Days in a row of Lean Mode journaling _____

lbs.

Met food goal today _____

- free day _____

Glasses of water _____

Su  M  Tu  W  Th  F  Sa  **Select Day of Week**

# Lean Mode Food Diary **Daily Page** FOR ___/___/___

| What I ate/drank | Where/When | Quantity | Calories | Fat Grams | Carbs Grams | Fiber Grams | Protein Grams | |
|---|---|---|---|---|---|---|---|---|
| | | | | | | | | |
| | | | | | | | | |
| | | | | | | | | |
| | | | | | | | | |
| | | | | | | | | |
| | | | | | | | | |
| | | | | | | | | |
| | | | | | | | | |
| | | | | | | | | |
| | | | | | | | | |
| | | | | | | | | |
| | | | | | | | | |
| | | | | | | | | |
| | | | | | | | | |
| **FOOD TOTALS:** | | | | | | | | |

**Color in** the FoodDots above that show healthy eating.
Try to connect-the-FoodDots with color.

| | Where | When | Duration | Distance | |
|---|---|---|---|---|---|
| Exercise | | | | | |
| | | | | | |
| **EXERCISE TOTALS:** | | | | | |

# Color in
## today's PowerCircles!

Met exercise goal today _____

Days in a row of
Lean Mode journaling _____          _____ lbs.

Met food goal today _____

- free day _____

Glasses of water _____

# Lean Mode Food Diary **Daily Page** FOR _____/_____/_____

| | What I ate/drank | Where/When | Quantity | Calories | Fat Grams | Carbs Grams | Fiber Grams | Protein Grams | |
|---|---|---|---|---|---|---|---|---|---|
| | | | | | | | | | |
| | | | | | | | | | |
| | | | | | | | | | |
| | | | | | | | | | |
| | | | | | | | | | |
| | | | | | | | | | |
| | | | | | | | | | |
| | | | | | | | | | |
| | | | | | | | | | |
| | | | | | | | | | |
| | | | | | | | | | |
| | | | | | | | | | |
| | | | | | | | | | |
| | **FOOD TOTALS:** | | | | | | | | |

**Color in** the FoodDots above that show healthy eating. Try to connect-the-FoodDots with color.

| | Where | When | Duration | Distance | |
|---|---|---|---|---|---|
| Exercise | | | | | |
| **EXERCISE TOTALS:** | | | | | |

# Color in
## today's PowerCircles!

Met exercise goal today _____

Met food goal today _____

Days in a row of Lean Mode journaling _____

_____ - free day

lbs.

Glasses of water _____

# Fill in Your **Color Code & Goals Page**

Take baby steps! Gradually build better habits by setting realistic goals here.

**NOTES:**

Set up your Goals and Color Code for the WEEK of ___ / ___ / ___ thru ___ / ___ / ___   Journaling Week # _____

| **DAILY GOALS** (Your choice of sections below) ○ Same as last week | **WEEKLY GOALS** ○ Same as last week | **WEEKLY TAB** Review your PowerCircles at week's end |
|---|---|---|
| **My daily food goal is:** _____ **calories** My color for meeting all my daily food goals: ( ) ( ) ( ) ( ) | I'll meet the goal at left at least _____ times per week | Did I meet my weekly goal at left? **YES,** I met my weekly goal! (Color it in) |
| **I'll include these healthy foods each day:** FoodDot Color    Food Group/Item    Amount _Optional Lean Mode Lite Day_ | I'll meet the goal at left at least _____ times per week _____ times per week _____ times per week | Did I meet my weekly goal at left? **YES,** I met my weekly goal! (Color it in) |
| **I'll color in a** _____ **- free day** (e.g. sugar-free, pastry-free, soda-free, etc.) in this color in this spot in my PowerCircles: | I'll meet the goal at left at least _____ times per week | Did I meet my weekly goal at left? **YES,** I met my weekly goal! (Color it in) |
| **My daily exercise goal is:** _____ My color for meeting my daily exercise goal is: | I'll meet the goal at left at least _____ times per week | Did I meet my weekly goal at left? **YES,** I met my weekly goal! (Color it in) |

My **4WEEK BUBBLE REWARD** for meeting all my weekly goals will be: _____

# Lean Mode Food Diary **Daily Page** FOR _____ / ____ / _____

| What I ate/drank | Where/When | Quantity | Calories | Fat Grams | Carbs Grams | Fiber Grams | Protein Grams |
|---|---|---|---|---|---|---|---|
| | | | | | | | |
| | | | | | | | |
| | | | | | | | |
| | | | | | | | |
| | | | | | | | |
| | | | | | | | |
| | | | | | | | |
| | | | | | | | |
| | | | | | | | |
| | | | | | | | |
| | | | | | | | |
| | | | | | | | |
| | | | | | | | |
| | | | | | | | |
| **FOOD TOTALS:** | | | | | | | |

**Color in** the FoodDots above that show healthy eating.
Try to connect-the-FoodDots with color.

| | Where | When | Duration | Distance |
|---|---|---|---|---|
| Exercise | | | | |
| **EXERCISE TOTALS:** | | | | |

## Color in today's PowerCircles!

Met exercise goal today _____

Days in a row of Lean Mode journaling _____    lbs.

Met food goal today _____

- free day _____

Glasses of water _____

Su M Tu W Th F Sa   Select Day of Week

# Lean Mode Food Diary **Daily Page** FOR ___ / ___ / ___

| What I ate/drank | Where/When | Quantity | Calories | Fat Grams | Carbs Grams | Fiber Grams | Protein Grams | |
|---|---|---|---|---|---|---|---|---|
| | | | | | | | | |
| | | | | | | | | |
| | | | | | | | | |
| | | | | | | | | |
| | | | | | | | | |
| | | | | | | | | |
| | | | | | | | | |
| | | | | | | | | |
| | | | | | | | | |
| | | | | | | | | |
| | | | | | | | | |
| | | | | | | | | |
| **FOOD TOTALS:** | | | | | | | | |

**Color in** the FoodDots above that show healthy eating.
Try to connect-the-FoodDots with color.

| | Where | When | Duration | Distance | |
|---|---|---|---|---|---|
| Exercise | | | | | |
| **EXERCISE TOTALS:** | | | | | |

## Color in today's PowerCircles!

Met exercise goal today ___

Days in a row of Lean Mode journaling ___

___ lbs.

Met food goal today ___

- free day ___

Glasses of water ___

Su M Tu W Th F Sa Select Day of Week

# Lean Mode Food Diary **Daily Page** FOR _____ / _____ / _____

| What I ate/drank | Where/When | Quantity | Calories | Fat Grams | Carbs Grams | Fiber Grams | Protein Grams | |
|---|---|---|---|---|---|---|---|---|
| | | | | | | | | |
| | | | | | | | | |
| | | | | | | | | |
| | | | | | | | | |
| | | | | | | | | |
| | | | | | | | | |
| | | | | | | | | |
| | | | | | | | | |
| | | | | | | | | |
| | | | | | | | | |
| | | | | | | | | |
| | | | | | | | | |
| | | | | | | | | |
| | | | | | | | | |
| **FOOD TOTALS:** | | | | | | | | |

**Color in** the FoodDots above that show healthy eating.
Try to connect-the-FoodDots with color.

| | Where | When | Duration | Distance | |
|---|---|---|---|---|---|
| Exercise | | | | | |
| **EXERCISE TOTALS:** | | | | | |

## Color in today's PowerCircles!

Met exercise goal today _____

Days in a row of Lean Mode journaling _____    lbs.

Met food goal today _____

- free day _____

Glasses of water _____

Su  M  Tu  W  Th  F  Sa   Select Day
of Week

# Lean Mode Food Diary **Daily Page** FOR ___ / ___ / ___

| What I ate/drank | Where/When | Quantity | Calories | Fat Grams | Carbs Grams | Fiber Grams | Protein Grams | |
|---|---|---|---|---|---|---|---|---|
| | | | | | | | | |
| | | | | | | | | |
| | | | | | | | | |
| | | | | | | | | |
| | | | | | | | | |
| | | | | | | | | |
| | | | | | | | | |
| | | | | | | | | |
| | | | | | | | | |
| | | | | | | | | |
| | | | | | | | | |
| | | | | | | | | |
| **FOOD TOTALS:** | | | | | | | | |

**Color in** the FoodDots above that show healthy eating.
Try to connect-the-FoodDots with color.

| | Where | When | Duration | Distance | | |
|---|---|---|---|---|---|---|
| Exercise | | | | | | |
| **EXERCISE TOTALS:** | | | | | | |

# Color in
## today's PowerCircles!

Met exercise goal today ........................

Days in a row of
Lean Mode journaling          lbs.

Met food goal today ........................

- free day

Glasses of water

# Lean Mode Food Diary **Daily Page** FOR _____ / _____ / _____

| What I ate/drank | Where/When | Quantity | Calories | Fat Grams | Carbs Grams | Fiber Grams | Protein Grams | |
|---|---|---|---|---|---|---|---|---|
| | | | | | | | | |
| | | | | | | | | |
| | | | | | | | | |
| | | | | | | | | |
| | | | | | | | | |
| | | | | | | | | |
| | | | | | | | | |
| | | | | | | | | |
| | | | | | | | | |
| | | | | | | | | |
| | | | | | | | | |
| | | | | | | | | |
| | | | | | | | | |
| **FOOD TOTALS:** | | | | | | | | |

**Color in** the FoodDots above that show healthy eating.
Try to connect-the-FoodDots with color.

| | Where | When | Duration | Distance | |
|---|---|---|---|---|---|
| Exercise | | | | | |
| **EXERCISE TOTALS:** | | | | | |

## Color in today's PowerCircles!

Met exercise goal today _____

Days in a row of
Lean Mode journaling _____

_____ lbs.

Met food goal today _____

- free day _____

Glasses of water _____

(Su) (M) (Tu) (W) (Th) (F) (Sa)  Select Day of Week

# Lean Mode Food Diary **Daily Page** FOR _____ / ___ / _____

| | What I ate/drank | Where/When | Quantity | Calories | Fat Grams | Carbs Grams | Fiber Grams | Protein Grams | |
|---|---|---|---|---|---|---|---|---|---|
| | | | | | | | | | |
| | | | | | | | | | |
| | | | | | | | | | |
| | | | | | | | | | |
| | | | | | | | | | |
| | | | | | | | | | |
| | | | | | | | | | |
| | | | | | | | | | |
| | | | | | | | | | |
| | | | | | | | | | |
| | | | | | | | | | |

**FOOD TOTALS:**

**Color in** the FoodDots above that show healthy eating.
Try to connect-the-FoodDots with color.

| | Where | When | Duration | Distance | |
|---|---|---|---|---|---|
| Exercise | | | | | |

**EXERCISE TOTALS:**

## Color in
## today's PowerCircles!

Met exercise goal today _____

Days in a row of
Lean Mode journaling _____    lbs.

Met food goal today _____

_____ - free day

Glasses of water _____

Su  M  Tu  W  Th  F  Sa   Select Day of Week

# Lean Mode Food Diary **Daily Page** FOR _____/_____/_____

| What I ate/drank | Where/When | Quantity | Calories | Fat Grams | Carbs Grams | Fiber Grams | Protein Grams | |
|---|---|---|---|---|---|---|---|---|
|  |  |  |  |  |  |  |  |  |
|  |  |  |  |  |  |  |  |  |
|  |  |  |  |  |  |  |  |  |
|  |  |  |  |  |  |  |  |  |
|  |  |  |  |  |  |  |  |  |
|  |  |  |  |  |  |  |  |  |
|  |  |  |  |  |  |  |  |  |
|  |  |  |  |  |  |  |  |  |
|  |  |  |  |  |  |  |  |  |
|  |  |  |  |  |  |  |  |  |
|  |  |  |  |  |  |  |  |  |
| **FOOD TOTALS:** |  |  |  |  |  |  |  |  |

**Color in** the FoodDots above that show healthy eating.
Try to connect-the-FoodDots with color.

| Exercise | Where | When | Duration | Distance | |
|---|---|---|---|---|---|
|  |  |  |  |  |  |
| **EXERCISE TOTALS:** |  |  |  |  |  |

## Color in
today's PowerCircles!

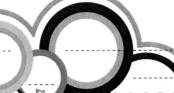

Met exercise goal today _____

Days in a row of
Lean Mode journaling _____     _____ lbs.

Met food goal today _____

- free day _____

Glasses of water _____

# Fill in Your **Color Code & Goals Page**

Take baby steps! Gradually build better habits by setting realistic goals here.

**NOTES:**

Set up your Goals and Color Code for the WEEK of ___/___/___ thru ___/___/___   Journaling Week # _____

| **DAILY GOALS** (Your choice of sections below)<br>○ Same as last week | **WEEKLY GOALS**<br>○ Same as last week | **WEEKLY TAB**<br>Review your PowerCircles at week's end |
|---|---|---|
| **My daily food goal is:** _____ **calories**<br>My color for meeting all my daily food goals:   (   )<br>(   )<br>(   )<br>(   ) | I'll meet the goal at left at least _____ times per week | Did I meet my weekly goal at left?   **YES,** I met my weekly goal!   (Color it in) |
| **I'll include these healthy foods each day:**<br>FoodDot Color   Food Group/Item   Amount<br>*Optional Lean Mode Lite Day* | I'll meet the goal at left at least<br>_____ times per week<br>_____ times per week<br>_____ times per week | Did I meet my weekly goal at left?   **YES,** I met my weekly goal!   (Color it in) |
| **I'll color in a _____ - free day**<br>(e.g. sugar-free, pastry-free, soda-free, etc.)<br>in this color in this spot in my PowerCircles: | I'll meet the goal at left at least _____ times per week | Did I meet my weekly goal at left?   **YES,** I met my weekly goal!   (Color it in) |
| **My daily exercise goal is:** _____<br>My color for meeting my daily exercise goal is: | I'll meet the goal at left at least _____ times per week | Did I meet my weekly goal at left?   **YES,** I met my weekly goal!   (Color it in) |

My **4WEEK BUBBLE REWARD** for meeting all my weekly goals will be: _____

# Lean Mode Food Diary **Daily Page** FOR _____ / _____ / _____

| What I ate/drank | Where/When | Quantity | Calories | Fat Grams | Carbs Grams | Fiber Grams | Protein Grams | |
|---|---|---|---|---|---|---|---|---|
| | | | | | | | | |
| | | | | | | | | |
| | | | | | | | | |
| | | | | | | | | |
| | | | | | | | | |
| | | | | | | | | |
| | | | | | | | | |
| | | | | | | | | |
| | | | | | | | | |
| | | | | | | | | |
| | | | | | | | | |
| | | | | | | | | |
| | | | | | | | | |
| | | | | | | | | |
| **FOOD TOTALS:** | | | | | | | | |

**Color in** the FoodDots above that show healthy eating.
Try to connect-the-FoodDots with color.

| | Where | When | Duration | Distance | |
|---|---|---|---|---|---|
| Exercise | | | | | |
| **EXERCISE TOTALS:** | | | | | |

## Color in today's PowerCircles!

Met exercise goal today _____

Days in a row of Lean Mode journaling _____

lbs.

Met food goal today _____

- free day _____

Glasses of water _____

# Lean Mode Food Diary **Daily Page** FOR _____ / _____ / _____

| What I ate/drank | Where/When | Quantity | Calories | Fat Grams | Carbs Grams | Fiber Grams | Protein Grams |
|---|---|---|---|---|---|---|---|
| | | | | | | | |
| | | | | | | | |
| | | | | | | | |
| | | | | | | | |
| | | | | | | | |
| | | | | | | | |
| | | | | | | | |
| | | | | | | | |
| | | | | | | | |
| | | | | | | | |
| | | | | | | | |
| | | | | | | | |
| **FOOD TOTALS:** | | | | | | | |

**Color in** the FoodDots above that show healthy eating.
Try to connect-the-FoodDots with color.

| | Where | When | Duration | Distance |
|---|---|---|---|---|
| Exercise | | | | |
| | | | | |
| **EXERCISE TOTALS:** | | | | |

## Color in today's PowerCircles!

Met exercise goal today _____

Met food goal today _____

Days in a row of Lean Mode journaling _____

lbs.

- free day _____

Glasses of water _____

Su  M  Tu  W  Th  F  Sa   Select Day of Week

# Lean Mode Food Diary **Daily Page** FOR _____ / _____ / _____

| | What I ate/drank | Where/When | Quantity | Calories | Fat Grams | Carbs Grams | Fiber Grams | Protein Grams |
|---|---|---|---|---|---|---|---|---|
| | | | | | | | | |
| | | | | | | | | |
| | | | | | | | | |
| | | | | | | | | |
| | | | | | | | | |
| | | | | | | | | |
| | | | | | | | | |
| | | | | | | | | |
| | | | | | | | | |
| | | | | | | | | |
| | | | | | | | | |
| | | | | | | | | |
| | | | | | | | | |
| | | | | | | | | |
| | **FOOD TOTALS:** | | | | | | | |

**Color in** the FoodDots above that show healthy eating.
Try to connect-the-FoodDots with color.

| | Where | When | Duration | Distance |
|---|---|---|---|---|
| Exercise | | | | |
| **EXERCISE TOTALS:** | | | | |

## Color in today's PowerCircles!

Met exercise goal today _____

Days in a row of Lean Mode journaling _____

_____ lbs.

Met food goal today _____

- free day _____

Glasses of water _____

# Lean Mode Food Diary **Daily Page** FOR _____ / _____ / _____

| | What I ate/drank | Where/When | Quantity | Calories | Fat Grams | Carbs Grams | Fiber Grams | Protein Grams |
|---|---|---|---|---|---|---|---|---|
| | | | | | | | | |
| | | | | | | | | |
| | | | | | | | | |
| | | | | | | | | |
| | | | | | | | | |
| | | | | | | | | |
| | | | | | | | | |
| | | | | | | | | |
| | | | | | | | | |
| | | | | | | | | |
| | | | | | | | | |
| | | | | | | | | |
| | | | | | | | | |
| | | | | | | | | |
| | **FOOD TOTALS:** | | | | | | | |

**Color in** the FoodDots above that show healthy eating.
Try to connect-the-FoodDots with color.

| | Where | When | Duration | Distance |
|---|---|---|---|---|
| Exercise | | | | |
| **EXERCISE TOTALS:** | | | | |

## Color in today's PowerCircles!

Met exercise goal today ..........

Days in a row of
Lean Mode journaling

lbs.

Met food goal today ..........

- free day

Glasses of water

Su  M  Tu  W  Th  F  Sa   Select Day
of Week

# Lean Mode Food Diary **Daily Page**  FOR _____ / _____ / _____

| What I ate/drank | Where/When | Quantity | Calories | Fat Grams | Carbs Grams | Fiber Grams | Protein Grams | |
|---|---|---|---|---|---|---|---|---|
| | | | | | | | | |
| | | | | | | | | |
| | | | | | | | | |
| | | | | | | | | |
| | | | | | | | | |
| | | | | | | | | |
| | | | | | | | | |
| | | | | | | | | |
| | | | | | | | | |
| | | | | | | | | |
| | | | | | | | | |
| | | | | | | | | |
| | | | | | | | | |
| | | | | | | | | |
| | | | | | | | | |
| **FOOD TOTALS:** | | | | | | | | |

**Color in** the FoodDots above that show healthy eating.
Try to connect-the-FoodDots with color.

| | Where | When | Duration | Distance | | |
|---|---|---|---|---|---|---|
| Exercise | | | | | | |
| **EXERCISE TOTALS:** | | | | | | |

## Color in
### today's PowerCircles!

Met exercise goal today _____

Days in a row of
Lean Mode journaling _____

lbs.

Met food goal today _____

- free day _____

Glasses of water _____

# Lean Mode Food Diary **Daily Page** FOR _____ / _____ / _____

| What I ate/drank | Where/When | Quantity | Calories | Fat Grams | Carbs Grams | Fiber Grams | Protein Grams | |
|---|---|---|---|---|---|---|---|---|
| | | | | | | | | |
| | | | | | | | | |
| | | | | | | | | |
| | | | | | | | | |
| | | | | | | | | |
| | | | | | | | | |
| | | | | | | | | |
| | | | | | | | | |
| | | | | | | | | |
| | | | | | | | | |
| | | | | | | | | |
| **FOOD TOTALS:** | | | | | | | | |

**Color in** the FoodDots above that show healthy eating.
Try to connect-the-FoodDots with color.

| | Where | When | Duration | Distance |
|---|---|---|---|---|
| Exercise | | | | |
| | | | | |
| **EXERCISE TOTALS:** | | | | |

## Color in today's PowerCircles!

Met exercise goal today _____

Days in a row of Lean Mode journaling _____

lbs.

Met food goal today _____

- free day _____

Glasses of water _____

Su  M  Tu  W  Th  F  Sa  Select Day of Week

# Lean Mode Food Diary **Daily Page**  FOR ___ / ___ / ___

| What I ate/drank | Where/When | Quantity | Calories | Fat Grams | Carbs Grams | Fiber Grams | Protein Grams | |
|---|---|---|---|---|---|---|---|---|
|  |  |  |  |  |  |  |  |  |
|  |  |  |  |  |  |  |  |  |
|  |  |  |  |  |  |  |  |  |
|  |  |  |  |  |  |  |  |  |
|  |  |  |  |  |  |  |  |  |
|  |  |  |  |  |  |  |  |  |
|  |  |  |  |  |  |  |  |  |
|  |  |  |  |  |  |  |  |  |
|  |  |  |  |  |  |  |  |  |
|  |  |  |  |  |  |  |  |  |
|  |  |  |  |  |  |  |  |  |
|  |  |  |  |  |  |  |  |  |
|  | **FOOD TOTALS:** |  |  |  |  |  |  |  |

**Color in** the FoodDots above that show healthy eating.
Try to connect-the-FoodDots with color.

| | Where | When | Duration | Distance | |
|---|---|---|---|---|---|
| Exercise |  |  |  |  |  |
|  | **EXERCISE TOTALS:** |  |  |  |  |

# Color in
## today's PowerCircles!

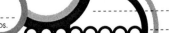

Met exercise goal today _____

Days in a row of
Lean Mode journaling _____          lbs.

Met food goal today _____

- free day _____

Glasses of water _____

# Fill in Your **Color Code & Goals Page**

Take baby steps! Gradually build better habits by setting realistic goals here.

**NOTES:**

Set up your Goals and Color Code for the WEEK of ___/___/___ thru ___/___/___   Journaling Week # _____

| **DAILY GOALS** (Your choice of sections below) ◯ Same as last week | **WEEKLY GOALS** ◯ Same as last week | **WEEKLY TAB** Review your PowerCircles at week's end |
|---|---|---|
| **My daily food goal is:** _____ **calories** My color for meeting all my daily food goals: ( ) ( ) ( ) ( ) | I'll meet the goal at left at least _____ times per week | Did I meet my weekly goal at left? **YES, I met my weekly goal!** (Color it in) |
| **I'll include these healthy foods each day:** FoodDot Color    Food Group/Item    Amount  Optional Lean Mode Lite Day | I'll meet the goal at left at least _____ times per week _____ times per week _____ times per week | Did I meet my weekly goal at left? **YES, I met my weekly goal!** (Color it in) |
| **I'll color in a** _____ **- free day** (e.g. sugar-free, pastry-free, soda-free, etc.) in this color in this spot in my PowerCircles: | I'll meet the goal at left at least _____ times per week | Did I meet my weekly goal at left? **YES, I met my weekly goal!** (Color it in) |
| **My daily exercise goal is:** _____ My color for meeting my daily exercise goal is: | I'll meet the goal at left at least _____ times per week | Did I meet my weekly goal at left? **YES, I met my weekly goal!** (Color it in) |

My **4WEEK BUBBLE REWARD** for meeting all my weekly goals will be: _____

Su  M  Tu  W  Th  F  Sa  Select Day of Week

# Lean Mode Food Diary **Daily Page** FOR _____ / ___ / ___

| | What I ate/drank | Where/When | Quantity | Calories | Fat Grams | Carbs Grams | Fiber Grams | Protein Grams | |
|---|---|---|---|---|---|---|---|---|---|
| | | | | | | | | | |
| | | | | | | | | | |
| | | | | | | | | | |
| | | | | | | | | | |
| | | | | | | | | | |
| | | | | | | | | | |
| | | | | | | | | | |
| | | | | | | | | | |
| | | | | | | | | | |
| | | | | | | | | | |
| | | | | | | | | | |
| | | | | | | | | | |
| | | | | | | | | | |
| | **FOOD TOTALS:** | | | | | | | | |

**Color in** the FoodDots above that show healthy eating.
Try to connect-the-FoodDots with color.

| | Where | When | Duration | Distance | | |
|---|---|---|---|---|---|---|
| Exercise | | | | | | |
| **EXERCISE TOTALS:** | | | | | | |

# Color in
## today's PowerCircles!

Met exercise goal today _____

Days in a row of Lean Mode journaling _____

lbs.

Met food goal today _____

- free day _____

Glasses of water _____

# Lean Mode Food Diary **Daily Page** FOR ____ / ____ / ____

| What I ate/drank | Where/When | Quantity | Calories | Fat Grams | Carbs Grams | Fiber Grams | Protein Grams |
|---|---|---|---|---|---|---|---|
| | | | | | | | |
| | | | | | | | |
| | | | | | | | |
| | | | | | | | |
| | | | | | | | |
| | | | | | | | |
| | | | | | | | |
| | | | | | | | |
| | | | | | | | |
| | | | | | | | |
| | | | | | | | |
| | | | | | | | |
| | | | | | | | |
| **FOOD TOTALS:** | | | | | | | |

**Color in** the FoodDots above that show healthy eating.
Try to connect-the-FoodDots with color.

| | Where | When | Duration | Distance |
|---|---|---|---|---|
| Exercise | | | | |
| **EXERCISE TOTALS:** | | | | |

## Color in today's PowerCircles!

Met exercise goal today ____

Days in a row of Lean Mode journaling ____

____ lbs.

Met food goal today ____

- free day ____

Glasses of water ____

# Lean Mode Food Diary **Daily Page** FOR ____ / ____ / ____

| What I ate/drank | Where/When | Quantity | Calories | Fat Grams | Carbs Grams | Fiber Grams | Protein Grams | |
|---|---|---|---|---|---|---|---|---|
| | | | | | | | | |
| | | | | | | | | |
| | | | | | | | | |
| | | | | | | | | |
| | | | | | | | | |
| | | | | | | | | |
| | | | | | | | | |
| | | | | | | | | |
| | | | | | | | | |
| | | | | | | | | |
| | | | | | | | | |
| | | | | | | | | |
| | | | | | | | | |
| **FOOD TOTALS:** | | | | | | | | |

**Color in** the FoodDots above that show healthy eating.
Try to connect-the-FoodDots with color.

| | Where | When | Duration | Distance |
|---|---|---|---|---|
| Exercise | | | | |
| **EXERCISE TOTALS:** | | | | |

## Color in today's PowerCircles!

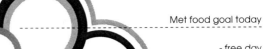

Met exercise goal today ................................................

Days in a row of
Lean Mode journaling ................................

Met food goal today ................................

- free day ................................

lbs.

Glasses of water

# Lean Mode Food Diary **Daily Page** FOR _____/_____/_____

| What I ate/drank | Where/When | Quantity | Calories | Fat Grams | Carbs Grams | Fiber Grams | Protein Grams | |
|---|---|---|---|---|---|---|---|---|
| | | | | | | | | |
| | | | | | | | | |
| | | | | | | | | |
| | | | | | | | | |
| | | | | | | | | |
| | | | | | | | | |
| | | | | | | | | |
| | | | | | | | | |
| | | | | | | | | |
| | | | | | | | | |
| | | | | | | | | |
| | | | | | | | | |
| **FOOD TOTALS:** | | | | | | | | |

**Color in** the FoodDots above that show healthy eating.
Try to connect-the-FoodDots with color.

| | Where | When | Duration | Distance | |
|---|---|---|---|---|---|
| Exercise | | | | | |
| **EXERCISE TOTALS:** | | | | | |

## Color in today's PowerCircles!

Met exercise goal today _____

Met food goal today _____

Days in a row of Lean Mode journaling _____

lbs. _____ - free day _____

Glasses of water _____

Su M Tu W Th F Sa  Select Day of Week

# Lean Mode Food Diary **Daily Page** FOR _____ / _____ / _____

| What I ate/drank | Where/When | Quantity | Calories | Fat Grams | Carbs Grams | Fiber Grams | Protein Grams | |
|---|---|---|---|---|---|---|---|---|
| | | | | | | | | |
| | | | | | | | | |
| | | | | | | | | |
| | | | | | | | | |
| | | | | | | | | |
| | | | | | | | | |
| | | | | | | | | |
| | | | | | | | | |
| | | | | | | | | |
| | | | | | | | | |
| **FOOD TOTALS:** | | | | | | | | |

**Color in** the FoodDots above that show healthy eating.
Try to connect-the-FoodDots with color.

| | Where | When | Duration | Distance | |
|---|---|---|---|---|---|
| Exercise | | | | | |
| **EXERCISE TOTALS:** | | | | | |

## Color in today's PowerCircles!

Met exercise goal today _____

Days in a row of Lean Mode journaling _____

lbs.

Met food goal today _____

- free day _____

Glasses of water

Su M Tu W Th F Sa  Select Day
of Week

# Lean Mode Food Diary **Daily Page** FOR _____ / _____ / _____

| What I ate/drank | Where/When | Quantity | Calories | Fat Grams | Carbs Grams | Fiber Grams | Protein Grams |
|---|---|---|---|---|---|---|---|
| | | | | | | | |
| | | | | | | | |
| | | | | | | | |
| | | | | | | | |
| | | | | | | | |
| | | | | | | | |
| | | | | | | | |
| | | | | | | | |
| | | | | | | | |
| | | | | | | | |
| | | | | | | | |
| | | | | | | | |
| | | | | | | | |
| | | | | | | | |
| **FOOD TOTALS:** | | | | | | | |

**Color in** the FoodDots above that show healthy eating.
Try to connect-the-FoodDots with color.

| | Where | When | Duration | Distance |
|---|---|---|---|---|
| Exercise | | | | |
| **EXERCISE TOTALS:** | | | | |

## Color in
### today's PowerCircles!

Met exercise goal today _____

Met food goal today _____

- free day _____

Days in a row of
Lean Mode journaling _____

lbs.

Glasses of water _____

# Lean Mode Food Diary **Daily Page**  FOR _____ / ____ / _____

| What I ate/drank | Where/When | Quantity | Calories | Fat Grams | Carbs Grams | Fiber Grams | Protein Grams | |
|---|---|---|---|---|---|---|---|---|
| | | | | | | | | |
| | | | | | | | | |
| | | | | | | | | |
| | | | | | | | | |
| | | | | | | | | |
| | | | | | | | | |
| | | | | | | | | |
| | | | | | | | | |
| | | | | | | | | |
| | | | | | | | | |
| | | | | | | | | |
| | | | | | | | | |
| | | | | | | | | |
| | | | | | | | | |
| | | | | | | | | |
| | | | | | | | | |
| **FOOD TOTALS:** | | | | | | | | |

**Color in** the FoodDots above that show healthy eating.
Try to connect-the-FoodDots with color.

| | Where | When | Duration | Distance |
|---|---|---|---|---|
| Exercise | | | | |
| **EXERCISE TOTALS:** | | | | |

## Color in
today's PowerCircles!

Met exercise goal today _____

Days in a row of
Lean Mode journaling _____    lbs.

Met food goal today _____

- free day _____

Glasses of water _____

# Complete Your **4Week Bubble**

Look back over your Weekly Tabs for the past 4 weeks and tally the results.

**4WEEK BUBBLE RECAP:** ___/___/___ thru ___/___/___
Start       End       +  or  –

| Weight | | | |
|--------|--|--|--|
| | | | |
| | | | |

**Yay!** I journaled every day

I journaled _____ days this period,
_____ days in a row this period,
and _____ days in a row to date.

The **REWARD** I gave myself for meeting all my weekly goals this period was:

_____
(Color in your **4WEEK BUBBLE** at right)

○ NO, I didn't meet all my weekly goals, but here's what I need to change to succeed next month:
_____

**YES,** I met ALL my weekly goals!

Set up your Goals and Color Code for the WEEK of ___/___/___ thru ___/___/___    Journaling Week # _____

| **DAILY GOALS** (Your choice of sections below)<br>○ Same as last week | **WEEKLY GOALS**<br>○ Same as last week | **WEEKLY TAB**<br>Review your PowerCircles at week's end |
|---|---|---|
| **My daily food goal is:** _____ **calories**<br>My color for meeting all my daily food goals:<br>(  )<br>(  )<br>(  )<br>(  ) | I'll meet the goal at left at least _____ times per week | Did I meet my weekly goal at left?    **YES,** I met my weekly goal!  (Color it in) |
| **I'll include these healthy foods each day:**<br>FoodDot Color    Food Group/Item    Amount<br><br>Optional Lean Mode Lite Day | I'll meet the goal at left at least<br>_____ times per week<br>_____ times per week<br>_____ times per week | Did I meet my weekly goal at left?    **YES,** I met my weekly goal!  (Color it in) |
| **I'll color in a** _____ **- free day**<br>(e.g. sugar-free, pastry-free, soda-free, etc.)<br>in this color in this spot in my PowerCircles: | I'll meet the goal at left at least _____ times per week | Did I meet my weekly goal at left?    **YES,** I met my weekly goal!  (Color it in) |
| **My daily exercise goal is:** _____<br>My color for meeting my daily exercise goal is: | I'll meet the goal at left at least _____ times per week | Did I meet my weekly goal at left?    **YES,** I met my weekly goal!  (Color it in) |

My **4WEEK BUBBLE REWARD** for meeting all my weekly goals will be: _____

Su M Tu W Th F Sa  Select Day of Week

# Lean Mode Food Diary **Daily Page** FOR _____ / _____ / _____

| What I ate/drank | Where/When | Quantity | Calories | Fat Grams | Carbs Grams | Fiber Grams | Protein Grams | |
|---|---|---|---|---|---|---|---|---|
| | | | | | | | | |
| | | | | | | | | |
| | | | | | | | | |
| | | | | | | | | |
| | | | | | | | | |
| | | | | | | | | |
| | | | | | | | | |
| | | | | | | | | |
| | | | | | | | | |
| | | | | | | | | |
| | | | | | | | | |
| **FOOD TOTALS:** | | | | | | | | |

**Color in** the FoodDots above that show healthy eating.
Try to connect-the-FoodDots with color.

| | Where | When | Duration | Distance | |
|---|---|---|---|---|---|
| Exercise | | | | | |
| **EXERCISE TOTALS:** | | | | | |

## Color in today's PowerCircles!

Met exercise goal today _____

Days in a row of Lean Mode journaling _____

lbs. ____

Met food goal today _____

- free day _____

Glasses of water _____

# Lean Mode Food Diary **Daily Page** FOR _____ / _____ / _____

| What I ate/drank | Where/When | Quantity | Calories | Fat Grams | Carbs Grams | Fiber Grams | Protein Grams | |
|---|---|---|---|---|---|---|---|---|
| | | | | | | | | |
| | | | | | | | | |
| | | | | | | | | |
| | | | | | | | | |
| | | | | | | | | |
| | | | | | | | | |
| | | | | | | | | |
| | | | | | | | | |
| | | | | | | | | |
| | | | | | | | | |
| | | | | | | | | |
| | | | | | | | | |
| | | | | | | | | |
| | | | | | | | | |
| | | | | | | | | |
| **FOOD TOTALS:** | | | | | | | | |

**Color in** the FoodDots above that show healthy eating.
Try to connect-the-FoodDots with color.

| | Where | When | Duration | Distance |
|---|---|---|---|---|
| Exercise | | | | |
| **EXERCISE TOTALS:** | | | | |

# Color in
## today's PowerCircles!

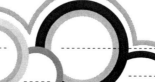

Met exercise goal today _____

Met food goal today _____

Days in a row of
Lean Mode journaling _____

_____ lbs.

- free day _____

Glasses of water _____

Su M Tu W Th F Sa Select Day of Week

# Lean Mode Food Diary **Daily Page** FOR _____/_____/_____

| What I ate/drank | Where/When | Quantity | Calories | Fat Grams | Carbs Grams | Fiber Grams | Protein Grams | |
|---|---|---|---|---|---|---|---|---|
| | | | | | | | | |
| | | | | | | | | |
| | | | | | | | | |
| | | | | | | | | |
| | | | | | | | | |
| | | | | | | | | |
| | | | | | | | | |
| | | | | | | | | |
| | | | | | | | | |
| | | | | | | | | |
| | | | | | | | | |
| | | | | | | | | |
| | | | | | | | | |
| | | | | | | | | |
| **FOOD TOTALS:** | | | | | | | | |

**Color in** the FoodDots above that show healthy eating.
Try to connect-the-FoodDots with color.

| | Where | When | Duration | Distance | |
|---|---|---|---|---|---|
| Exercise | | | | | |
| **EXERCISE TOTALS:** | | | | | |

## Color in
today's PowerCircles!

Met exercise goal today _____

Days in a row of
Lean Mode journaling _____

lbs.

Met food goal today _____

- free day _____

Glasses of water _____

# Lean Mode Food Diary **Daily Page** FOR ___ / ___ / ___

| | What I ate/drank | Where/When | Quantity | Calories | Fat Grams | Carbs Grams | Fiber Grams | Protein Grams | |
|---|---|---|---|---|---|---|---|---|---|
| | | | | | | | | | |
| | | | | | | | | | |
| | | | | | | | | | |
| | | | | | | | | | |
| | | | | | | | | | |
| | | | | | | | | | |
| | | | | | | | | | |
| | | | | | | | | | |
| | | | | | | | | | |
| | | | | | | | | | |
| | | | | | | | | | |
| | **FOOD TOTALS:** | | | | | | | | |

**Color in** the FoodDots above that show healthy eating.
Try to connect-the-FoodDots with color.

| | Where | When | Duration | Distance | |
|---|---|---|---|---|---|
| Exercise | | | | | |
| **EXERCISE TOTALS:** | | | | | |

## Color in today's PowerCircles!

Met exercise goal today ___

Met food goal today ___

Days in a row of Lean Mode journaling ___

___ lbs.

- free day ___

Glasses of water ___

# Lean Mode Food Diary **Daily Page**  FOR _____ / _____ / _____

| What I ate/drank | Where/When | Quantity | Calories | Fat Grams | Carbs Grams | Fiber Grams | Protein Grams |
|---|---|---|---|---|---|---|---|
| | | | | | | | |
| | | | | | | | |
| | | | | | | | |
| | | | | | | | |
| | | | | | | | |
| | | | | | | | |
| | | | | | | | |
| | | | | | | | |
| | | | | | | | |
| | | | | | | | |
| | | | | | | | |
| | | | | | | | |
| | | | | | | | |
| **FOOD TOTALS:** | | | | | | | |

**Color in** the FoodDots above that show healthy eating.
Try to connect-the-FoodDots with color.

| | Where | When | Duration | Distance | |
|---|---|---|---|---|---|
| Exercise | | | | | |
| **EXERCISE TOTALS:** | | | | | |

## Color in today's PowerCircles!

Met exercise goal today _____

Days in a row of Lean Mode journaling _____

_____ lbs.

Met food goal today _____

- free day _____

Glasses of water _____

# Lean Mode Food Diary **Daily Page** FOR ___ / ___ / ___

| What I ate/drank | Where/When | Quantity | Calories | Fat Grams | Carbs Grams | Fiber Grams | Protein Grams | |
|---|---|---|---|---|---|---|---|---|
| | | | | | | | | |

**FOOD TOTALS:**

**Color in** the FoodDots above that show healthy eating.
Try to connect-the-FoodDots with color.

| | Where | When | Duration | Distance | |
|---|---|---|---|---|---|
| Exercise | | | | | |

**EXERCISE TOTALS:**

## Color in today's PowerCircles!

Met exercise goal today ____

Days in a row of Lean Mode journaling ____    lbs.

Met food goal today ____

- free day ____

Glasses of water ____

Su  M  Tu  W  Th  F  Sa   Select Day
of Week

# Lean Mode Food Diary **Daily Page**   FOR ____ / ____ / ____

| What I ate/drank | Where/When | Quantity | Calories | Fat Grams | Carbs Grams | Fiber Grams | Protein Grams | |
|---|---|---|---|---|---|---|---|---|
| | | | | | | | | |
| | | | | | | | | |
| | | | | | | | | |
| | | | | | | | | |
| | | | | | | | | |
| | | | | | | | | |
| | | | | | | | | |
| | | | | | | | | |
| | | | | | | | | |
| | | | | | | | | |
| | | | | | | | | |
| | | | | | | | | |
| **FOOD TOTALS:** | | | | | | | | |

**Color in** the FoodDots above that show healthy eating.
Try to connect-the-FoodDots with color.

| | Where | When | Duration | Distance | |
|---|---|---|---|---|---|
| Exercise | | | | | |
| **EXERCISE TOTALS:** | | | | | |

## Color in
### today's PowerCircles!

Met exercise goal today _____

Met food goal today _____

- free day _____

Days in a row of
Lean Mode journaling _____

lbs.

Glasses of water _____

# Fill in Your **Color Code & Goals Page**

Take baby steps! Gradually build better habits by setting realistic goals here.

**NOTES:**

Set up your Goals and Color Code for the WEEK of ___/___/___ thru ___/___/___    Journaling Week # _____

| DAILY GOALS (Your choice of sections below) ◯ Same as last week | WEEKLY GOALS ◯ Same as last week | WEEKLY TAB Review your PowerCircles at week's end |
|---|---|---|
| **My daily food goal is:** _____ **calories**  My color for meeting all my daily food goals:  (    )  (    )  (    )  (    ) | I'll meet the goal at left at least _____ times per week | Did I meet my weekly goal at left?  **YES,** I met my weekly goal! (Color it in) |
| **I'll include these healthy foods each day:** FoodDot Color    Food Group/Item    Amount  Optional Lean Mode Lite Day | I'll meet the goal at left at least _____ times per week _____ times per week _____ times per week | Did I meet my weekly goal at left?  **YES,** I met my weekly goal! (Color it in) |
| **I'll color in a** _____ **- free day** (e.g. sugar-free, pastry-free, soda-free, etc.)  in this color in this spot in my PowerCircles: | I'll meet the goal at left at least _____ times per week | Did I meet my weekly goal at left?  **YES,** I met my weekly goal! (Color it in) |
| **My daily exercise goal is:** _____  My color for meeting my daily exercise goal is: | I'll meet the goal at left at least _____ times per week | Did I meet my weekly goal at left?  **YES,** I met my weekly goal! (Color it in) |

My **4WEEK BUBBLE REWARD** for meeting all my weekly goals will be: _____

Su  M  Tu  W  Th  F  Sa    Select Day of Week

# Lean Mode Food Diary **Daily Page**  FOR _____ / _____ / _____

| | What I ate/drank | Where/When | Quantity | Calories | Fat Grams | Carbs Grams | Fiber Grams | Protein Grams | |
|---|---|---|---|---|---|---|---|---|---|
| | | | | | | | | | |
| | | | | | | | | | |
| | | | | | | | | | |
| | | | | | | | | | |
| | | | | | | | | | |
| | | | | | | | | | |
| | | | | | | | | | |
| | | | | | | | | | |
| | | | | | | | | | |
| | | | | | | | | | |
| | | | | | | | | | |
| | | | | | | | | | |
| | | **FOOD TOTALS:** | | | | | | | |

**Color in** the FoodDots above that show healthy eating.
Try to connect-the-FoodDots with color.

| | Where | When | Duration | Distance | |
|---|---|---|---|---|---|
| Exercise | | | | | |
| | **EXERCISE TOTALS:** | | | | |

# Color in
## today's PowerCircles!

Met exercise goal today ........................................

Days in a row of
Lean Mode journaling ...............

_____ lbs.

Met food goal today ...............

- free day

Glasses of water

Su M Tu W Th F Sa  **Select Day of Week**

# Lean Mode Food Diary **Daily Page** FOR ___ / ___ / ___

| What I ate/drank | Where/When | Quantity | Calories | Fat Grams | Carbs Grams | Fiber Grams | Protein Grams |
|---|---|---|---|---|---|---|---|
| | | | | | | | |
| | | | | | | | |
| | | | | | | | |
| | | | | | | | |
| | | | | | | | |
| | | | | | | | |
| | | | | | | | |
| | | | | | | | |
| | | | | | | | |
| | | | | | | | |
| | | | | | | | |
| | | | | | | | |
| | | | | | | | |
| | | | | | | | |
| | | | | | | | |
| | | | | | | | |
| | | | | | | | |
| | | | | | | | |
| **FOOD TOTALS:** | | | | | | | |

**Color in** the FoodDots above that show healthy eating.
Try to connect-the-FoodDots with color.

| | Where | When | Duration | Distance |
|---|---|---|---|---|
| Exercise | | | | |
| | | | | |
| **EXERCISE TOTALS:** | | | | |

# Color in
## today's PowerCircles!

Met exercise goal today ___

Days in a row of
Lean Mode journaling ___

___ lbs.

Met food goal today ___

- free day ___

Glasses of water ___

# Lean Mode Food Diary **Daily Page** FOR _____ / _____ / _____

| What I ate/drank | Where/When | Quantity | Calories | Fat Grams | Carbs Grams | Fiber Grams | Protein Grams | |
|---|---|---|---|---|---|---|---|---|
| | | | | | | | | |
| | | | | | | | | |
| | | | | | | | | |
| | | | | | | | | |
| | | | | | | | | |
| | | | | | | | | |
| | | | | | | | | |
| | | | | | | | | |
| | | | | | | | | |
| | | | | | | | | |
| | | | | | | | | |
| | | | | | | | | |
| **FOOD TOTALS:** | | | | | | | | |

**Color in** the FoodDots above that show healthy eating. Try to connect-the-FoodDots with color.

| | Where | When | Duration | Distance | |
|---|---|---|---|---|---|
| Exercise | | | | | |
| **EXERCISE TOTALS:** | | | | | |

## Color in today's PowerCircles!

Met exercise goal today _____

Days in a row of Lean Mode journaling _____

lbs.

Met food goal today _____

- free day _____

Glasses of water _____

Su  M  Tu  W  Th  F  Sa    Select Day
                           of Week

# Lean Mode Food Diary **Daily Page** FOR _____ / _____ / _____

| What I ate/drank | Where/When | Quantity | Calories | Fat Grams | Carbs Grams | Fiber Grams | Protein Grams |
|---|---|---|---|---|---|---|---|
| | | | | | | | |
| | | | | | | | |
| | | | | | | | |
| | | | | | | | |
| | | | | | | | |
| | | | | | | | |
| | | | | | | | |
| | | | | | | | |
| | | | | | | | |
| | | | | | | | |
| | | | | | | | |
| | | | | | | | |
| | | | | | | | |
| | | | | | | | |
| **FOOD TOTALS:** | | | | | | | |

**Color in** the FoodDots above that show healthy eating.
Try to connect-the-FoodDots with color.

| | Where | When | Duration | Distance |
|---|---|---|---|---|
| Exercise | | | | |
| **EXERCISE TOTALS:** | | | | |

## Color in
today's PowerCircles!

Met exercise goal today _____

Days in a row of
Lean Mode journaling _____    _____ lbs.

Met food goal today _____

_____ - free day

Glasses of water _____

Su  M  Tu  W  Th  F  Sa  Select Day of Week

# Lean Mode Food Diary **Daily Page** FOR _____ / _____ / _____

| What I ate/drank | Where/When | Quantity | Calories | Fat Grams | Carbs Grams | Fiber Grams | Protein Grams | |
|---|---|---|---|---|---|---|---|---|
| | | | | | | | | |
| | | | | | | | | |
| | | | | | | | | |
| | | | | | | | | |
| | | | | | | | | |
| | | | | | | | | |
| | | | | | | | | |
| | | | | | | | | |
| | | | | | | | | |
| | | | | | | | | |
| | | | | | | | | |
| | | | | | | | | |
| | | | | | | | | |
| | | | | | | | | |
| **FOOD TOTALS:** | | | | | | | | |

**Color in** the FoodDots above that show healthy eating.
Try to connect-the-FoodDots with color.

| | Where | When | Duration | Distance | |
|---|---|---|---|---|---|
| Exercise | | | | | |
| **EXERCISE TOTALS:** | | | | | |

## Color in today's PowerCircles!

Met exercise goal today _____

Met food goal today _____

- free day _____

Days in a row of Lean Mode journaling _____

lbs.

Glasses of water _____

# Lean Mode Food Diary **Daily Page** FOR _____ / _____ / _____

| What I ate/drank | Where/When | Quantity | Calories | Fat Grams | Carbs Grams | Fiber Grams | Protein Grams |
|---|---|---|---|---|---|---|---|
| | | | | | | | |
| | | | | | | | |
| | | | | | | | |
| | | | | | | | |
| | | | | | | | |
| | | | | | | | |
| | | | | | | | |
| | | | | | | | |
| | | | | | | | |
| | | | | | | | |
| | | | | | | | |
| | | | | | | | |
| | | | | | | | |
| **FOOD TOTALS:** | | | | | | | |

**Color in** the FoodDots above that show healthy eating.
Try to connect-the-FoodDots with color.

| | Where | When | Duration | Distance |
|---|---|---|---|---|
| Exercise | | | | |
| **EXERCISE TOTALS:** | | | | |

## Color in today's PowerCircles!

Met exercise goal today _____

Days in a row of Lean Mode journaling _____

_____ lbs.

Met food goal today _____

_____ - free day

Glasses of water _____

Su  M  Tu  W  Th  F  Sa    Select Day
of Week

# Lean Mode Food Diary **Daily Page**    FOR _____ / _____ / _____

| What I ate/drank | Where/When | Quantity | Calories | Fat Grams | Carbs Grams | Fiber Grams | Protein Grams |
|---|---|---|---|---|---|---|---|
| | | | | | | | |
| | | | | | | | |
| | | | | | | | |
| | | | | | | | |
| | | | | | | | |
| | | | | | | | |
| | | | | | | | |
| | | | | | | | |
| | | | | | | | |
| | | | | | | | |
| | | | | | | | |
| | | | | | | | |
| | | | | | | | |
| | | | | | | | |
| **FOOD TOTALS:** | | | | | | | |

**Color in** the FoodDots above that show healthy eating.
Try to connect-the-FoodDots with color.

| | Where | When | Duration | Distance |
|---|---|---|---|---|
| Exercise | | | | |
| **EXERCISE TOTALS:** | | | | |

## Color in
### today's PowerCircles!

Met exercise goal today _____

Days in a row of
Lean Mode journaling _____

_____ lbs.

Met food goal today _____

- free day _____

Glasses of water _____

# Fill in Your **Color Code & Goals Page**

Take baby steps! Gradually build better habits by setting realistic goals here.

**NOTES:**

Set up your Goals and Color Code for the WEEK of ___/___/___ thru ___/___/___ Journaling Week # _____

| **DAILY GOALS** (Your choice of sections below) ○ Same as last week | **WEEKLY GOALS** ○ Same as last week | **WEEKLY TAB** Review your PowerCircles at week's end |
|---|---|---|
| **My daily food goal is:** _____ **calories** My color for meeting all my daily food goals: ( ) ( ) ( ) ( ) | I'll meet the goal at left at least _____ times per week | Did I meet my weekly goal at left? **YES,** I met my weekly goal! (Color it in) |
| **I'll include these healthy foods each day:** FoodDot Color    Food Group/Item    Amount Optional Lean Mode Lite Day | I'll meet the goal at left at least _____ times per week _____ times per week _____ times per week | Did I meet my weekly goal at left? **YES,** I met my weekly goal! (Color it in) |
| **I'll color in a** _____ **- free day** (e.g. sugar-free, pastry-free, soda-free, etc.) in this color in this spot in my PowerCircles: | I'll meet the goal at left at least _____ times per week | Did I meet my weekly goal at left? **YES,** I met my weekly goal! (Color it in) |
| **My daily exercise goal is:** _____ My color for meeting my daily exercise goal is: | I'll meet the goal at left at least _____ times per week | Did I meet my weekly goal at left? **YES,** I met my weekly goal! (Color it in) |

My **4WEEK BUBBLE REWARD** for meeting all my weekly goals will be: _____

# Lean Mode Food Diary **Daily Page** FOR ____ / ____ / ____

| What I ate/drank | Where/When | Quantity | Calories | Fat Grams | Carbs Grams | Fiber Grams | Protein Grams | |
|---|---|---|---|---|---|---|---|---|
| | | | | | | | | |
| | | | | | | | | |
| | | | | | | | | |
| | | | | | | | | |
| | | | | | | | | |
| | | | | | | | | |
| | | | | | | | | |
| | | | | | | | | |
| | | | | | | | | |
| | | | | | | | | |
| | | | | | | | | |
| | | | | | | | | |
| | | | | | | | | |
| **FOOD TOTALS:** | | | | | | | | |

**Color in** the FoodDots above that show healthy eating.
Try to connect-the-FoodDots with color.

| | Where | When | Duration | Distance | | |
|---|---|---|---|---|---|---|
| Exercise | | | | | | |
| **EXERCISE TOTALS:** | | | | | | |

## Color in
### today's PowerCircles!

Met exercise goal today ____

Met food goal today ____

- free day ____

Days in a row of
Lean Mode journaling ____        lbs. ____        Glasses of water ____

# Lean Mode Food Diary **Daily Page** FOR ___/___/___

| What I ate/drank | Where/When | Quantity | Calories | Fat Grams | Carbs Grams | Fiber Grams | Protein Grams | |
|---|---|---|---|---|---|---|---|---|
| | | | | | | | | |
| | | | | | | | | |
| | | | | | | | | |
| | | | | | | | | |
| | | | | | | | | |
| | | | | | | | | |
| | | | | | | | | |
| | | | | | | | | |
| | | | | | | | | |
| | | | | | | | | |
| | | | | | | | | |
| | | | | | | | | |
| **FOOD TOTALS:** | | | | | | | | |

**Color in** the FoodDots above that show healthy eating.
Try to connect-the-FoodDots with color.

| | Where | When | Duration | Distance | |
|---|---|---|---|---|---|
| Exercise | | | | | |
| **EXERCISE TOTALS:** | | | | | |

# Color in today's PowerCircles!

Met exercise goal today ____

Days in a row of Lean Mode journaling ____

____ lbs.

Met food goal today ____

____ - free day

Glasses of water ____

Su M Tu W Th F Sa Select Day of Week

# Lean Mode Food Diary **Daily Page** FOR ___ / ___ / ___

| What I ate/drank | Where/When | Quantity | Calories | Fat Grams | Carbs Grams | Fiber Grams | Protein Grams |
|---|---|---|---|---|---|---|---|
| | | | | | | | |
| | | | | | | | |
| | | | | | | | |
| | | | | | | | |
| | | | | | | | |
| | | | | | | | |
| | | | | | | | |
| | | | | | | | |
| | | | | | | | |
| | | | | | | | |
| | | | | | | | |
| | | | | | | | |
| | | | | | | | |
| **FOOD TOTALS:** | | | | | | | |

**Color in** the FoodDots above that show healthy eating.
Try to connect-the-FoodDots with color.

| | Where | When | Duration | Distance |
|---|---|---|---|---|
| Exercise | | | | |
| **EXERCISE TOTALS:** | | | | |

## Color in today's PowerCircles!

Met exercise goal today _____

Days in a row of Lean Mode journaling _____

lbs.

Met food goal today _____

- free day _____

Glasses of water _____

Su M Tu W Th F Sa  **Select Day of Week**

# Lean Mode Food Diary **Daily Page** FOR _____ / _____ / _____

| What I ate/drank | Where/When | Quantity | Calories | Fat Grams | Carbs Grams | Fiber Grams | Protein Grams | |
|---|---|---|---|---|---|---|---|---|
| | | | | | | | | |
| | | | | | | | | |
| | | | | | | | | |
| | | | | | | | | |
| | | | | | | | | |
| | | | | | | | | |
| | | | | | | | | |
| | | | | | | | | |
| | | | | | | | | |
| | | | | | | | | |
| | | | | | | | | |
| | | | | | | | | |
| **FOOD TOTALS:** | | | | | | | | |

**Color in** the FoodDots above that show healthy eating.
Try to connect-the-FoodDots with color.

| | Where | When | Duration | Distance |
|---|---|---|---|---|
| Exercise | | | | |
| **EXERCISE TOTALS:** | | | | |

## Color in today's PowerCircles!

Met exercise goal today _____

Met food goal today _____

Days in a row of Lean Mode journaling _____

lbs.

- free day _____

Glasses of water _____

# Lean Mode Food Diary **Daily Page**  FOR _____ / _____ / _____

| What I ate/drank | Where/When | Quantity | Calories | Fat Grams | Carbs Grams | Fiber Grams | Protein Grams | |
|---|---|---|---|---|---|---|---|---|
| | | | | | | | | |
| | | | | | | | | |
| | | | | | | | | |
| | | | | | | | | |
| | | | | | | | | |
| | | | | | | | | |
| | | | | | | | | |
| | | | | | | | | |
| | | | | | | | | |
| | | | | | | | | |
| | | | | | | | | |
| | | | | | | | | |
| | | | | | | | | |
| **FOOD TOTALS:** | | | | | | | | |

**Color in** the FoodDots above that show healthy eating.
Try to connect-the-FoodDots with color.

| | Where | When | Duration | Distance | |
|---|---|---|---|---|---|
| Exercise | | | | | |
| **EXERCISE TOTALS:** | | | | | |

## Color in
today's PowerCircles!

Met exercise goal today _____

Days in a row of
Lean Mode journaling _____

lbs.

Met food goal today _____

- free day _____

Glasses of water _____

Su M Tu W Th F Sa **Select Day of Week**

# Lean Mode Food Diary **Daily Page** FOR _____ / _____ / _____

| | What I ate/drank | Where/When | Quantity | Calories | Fat Grams | Carbs Grams | Fiber Grams | Protein Grams |
|---|---|---|---|---|---|---|---|---|
| | | | | | | | | |
| | | | | | | | | |
| | | | | | | | | |
| | | | | | | | | |
| | | | | | | | | |
| | | | | | | | | |
| | | | | | | | | |
| | | | | | | | | |
| | | | | | | | | |
| | | | | | | | | |
| | | | | | | | | |
| | | | | | | | | |
| | | | | | | | | |
| | | | | | | | | |
| | | | | | | | | |
| | | | | | | | | |
| | **FOOD TOTALS:** | | | | | | | |

**Color in** the FoodDots above that show healthy eating.
Try to connect-the-FoodDots with color.

| | Where | When | Duration | Distance |
|---|---|---|---|---|
| Exercise | | | | |
| | | | | |
| | | | | |
| **EXERCISE TOTALS:** | | | | |

## Color in today's PowerCircles!

Met exercise goal today _____

Days in a row of _____
Lean Mode journaling

_____ lbs.

Met food goal today _____

_____ - free day

Glasses of water _____

Su  M  Tu  W  Th  F  Sa   Select Day
of Week

# Lean Mode Food Diary **Daily Page** FOR _____ / ___ / _____

| What I ate/drank | Where/When | Quantity | Calories | Fat Grams | Carbs Grams | Fiber Grams | Protein Grams | |
|---|---|---|---|---|---|---|---|---|
| | | | | | | | | |
| | | | | | | | | |
| | | | | | | | | |
| | | | | | | | | |
| | | | | | | | | |
| | | | | | | | | |
| | | | | | | | | |
| | | | | | | | | |
| | | | | | | | | |
| | | | | | | | | |
| | | | | | | | | |
| | | | | | | | | |
| | | | | | | | | |
| **FOOD TOTALS:** | | | | | | | | |

**Color in** the FoodDots above that show healthy eating.
Try to connect-the-FoodDots with color.

| | Where | When | Duration | Distance | |
|---|---|---|---|---|---|
| Exercise | | | | | |
| | | | | | |
| **EXERCISE TOTALS:** | | | | | |

## Color in
today's PowerCircles!

Met exercise goal today _____

Days in a row of
Lean Mode journaling _____

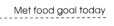
lbs.

Met food goal today _____

- free day _____

Glasses of water _____

# Fill in Your **Color Code & Goals Page**

Take baby steps! Gradually build better habits by setting realistic goals here.

**NOTES:**

Set up your Goals and Color Code for the WEEK of _ _ _ _/_ _ _/_ _ _ _ thru _ _ _ _/_ _ _/_ _ _ _ Journaling Week # _ _ _ _ _ _

| **DAILY GOALS** (Your choice of sections below) ○ Same as last week | **WEEKLY GOALS** ○ Same as last week | **WEEKLY TAB** Review your PowerCircles at week's end |
|---|---|---|
| **My daily food goal is:** _____ **calories** My color for meeting all my daily food goals: _____ ( ) _____ ( ) _____ ( ) _____ ( ) | I'll meet the goal at left at least _____ times per week | Did I meet my weekly goal at left? **YES, I met my weekly goal!** (Color it in) |
| **I'll include these healthy foods each day:** FoodDot Color   Food Group/Item   Amount *Optional Lean Mode Lite Day* | I'll meet the goal at left at least _____ times per week _____ times per week _____ times per week | Did I meet my weekly goal at left? **YES, I met my weekly goal!** (Color it in) |
| **I'll color in a** _____ **- free day** (e.g. sugar-free, pastry-free, soda-free, etc.) in this color in this spot in my PowerCircles: | I'll meet the goal at left at least _____ times per week | Did I meet my weekly goal at left? **YES, I met my weekly goal!** (Color it in) |
| **My daily exercise goal is:** _____ My color for meeting my daily exercise goal is: | I'll meet the goal at left at least _____ times per week | Did I meet my weekly goal at left? **YES, I met my weekly goal!** (Color it in) |

My **4WEEK BUBBLE REWARD** for meeting all my weekly goals will be: _____

Su  M  Tu  W  Th  F  Sa   Select Day of Week

# Lean Mode Food Diary **Daily Page** FOR _____ / _____ / _____

| What I ate/drank | Where/When | Quantity | Calories | Fat Grams | Carbs Grams | Fiber Grams | Protein Grams | |
|---|---|---|---|---|---|---|---|---|
| | | | | | | | | |
| | | | | | | | | |
| | | | | | | | | |
| | | | | | | | | |
| | | | | | | | | |
| | | | | | | | | |
| | | | | | | | | |
| | | | | | | | | |
| | | | | | | | | |
| | | | | | | | | |
| | | | | | | | | |
| **FOOD TOTALS:** | | | | | | | | |

**Color in** the FoodDots above that show healthy eating.
Try to connect-the-FoodDots with color.

| | Where | When | Duration | Distance | |
|---|---|---|---|---|---|
| Exercise | | | | | |
| **EXERCISE TOTALS:** | | | | | |

## Color in
### today's PowerCircles!

Met exercise goal today _____

Days in a row of
Lean Mode journaling _____

Met food goal today _____

- free day _____

lbs. _____

Glasses of water _____

Su  M  Tu  W  Th  F  Sa   Select Day
of Week

# Lean Mode Food Diary **Daily Page** FOR _____ / _____ / _____

| What I ate/drank | Where/When | Quantity | Calories | Fat Grams | Carbs Grams | Fiber Grams | Protein Grams | |
|---|---|---|---|---|---|---|---|---|
| | | | | | | | | |
| | | | | | | | | |
| | | | | | | | | |
| | | | | | | | | |
| | | | | | | | | |
| | | | | | | | | |
| | | | | | | | | |
| | | | | | | | | |
| | | | | | | | | |
| | | | | | | | | |
| | | | | | | | | |
| | | | | | | | | |
| **FOOD TOTALS:** | | | | | | | | |

**Color in** the FoodDots above that show healthy eating.
Try to connect-the-FoodDots with color.

| | Where | When | Duration | Distance |
|---|---|---|---|---|
| Exercise | | | | |
| **EXERCISE TOTALS:** | | | | |

# Color in
## today's PowerCircles!

Met exercise goal today _____

Days in a row of
Lean Mode journaling _____

_____ lbs.

Met food goal today _____

- free day _____

Glasses of water _____

Su  M  Tu  W  Th  F  Sa    Select Day of Week

# Lean Mode Food Diary **Daily Page** FOR ____ / ____ / ____

| What I ate/drank | Where/When | Quantity | Calories | Fat Grams | Carbs Grams | Fiber Grams | Protein Grams | |
|---|---|---|---|---|---|---|---|---|
| | | | | | | | | |
| | | | | | | | | |
| | | | | | | | | |
| | | | | | | | | |
| | | | | | | | | |
| | | | | | | | | |
| | | | | | | | | |
| | | | | | | | | |
| | | | | | | | | |
| | | | | | | | | |
| | | | | | | | | |
| | | | | | | | | |
| | | | | | | | | |
| **FOOD TOTALS:** | | | | | | | | |

**Color in** the FoodDots above that show healthy eating.
Try to connect-the-FoodDots with color.

| | Where | When | Duration | Distance | |
|---|---|---|---|---|---|
| Exercise | | | | | |
| **EXERCISE TOTALS:** | | | | | |

## Color in today's PowerCircles!

Met exercise goal today .................

Met food goal today .................

- free day

Days in a row of
Lean Mode journaling .................     lbs.

Glasses of water

Su M Tu W Th F Sa   **Select Day of Week**

# Lean Mode Food Diary **Daily Page** FOR ___ / ___ / ___

| What I ate/drank | Where/When | Quantity | Calories | Fat Grams | Carbs Grams | Fiber Grams | Protein Grams |
|---|---|---|---|---|---|---|---|
| | | | | | | | |
| | | | | | | | |
| | | | | | | | |
| | | | | | | | |
| | | | | | | | |
| | | | | | | | |
| | | | | | | | |
| | | | | | | | |
| | | | | | | | |
| | | | | | | | |
| | | | | | | | |
| | | | | | | | |
| | | | | | | | |
| **FOOD TOTALS:** | | | | | | | |

**Color in** the FoodDots above that show healthy eating.
Try to connect-the-FoodDots with color.

| | Where | When | Duration | Distance |
|---|---|---|---|---|
| Exercise | | | | |
| **EXERCISE TOTALS:** | | | | |

## Color in today's PowerCircles!

Met exercise goal today ___

Days in a row of Lean Mode journaling ___

___ lbs.

Met food goal today ___

- free day ___

Glasses of water ___

# Lean Mode Food Diary **Daily Page**    FOR _____ / _____ / _____

| What I ate/drank | Where/When | Quantity | Calories | Fat Grams | Carbs Grams | Fiber Grams | Protein Grams | |
|---|---|---|---|---|---|---|---|---|
| | | | | | | | | |
| | | | | | | | | |
| | | | | | | | | |
| | | | | | | | | |
| | | | | | | | | |
| | | | | | | | | |
| | | | | | | | | |
| | | | | | | | | |
| | | | | | | | | |
| | | | | | | | | |
| | | | | | | | | |
| | | | | | | | | |
| | | | | | | | | |
| **FOOD TOTALS:** | | | | | | | | |

**Color in** the FoodDots above that show healthy eating.
Try to connect-the-FoodDots with color.

| | Where | When | Duration | Distance | |
|---|---|---|---|---|---|
| Exercise | | | | | |
| **EXERCISE TOTALS:** | | | | | |

## Color in
today's PowerCircles!

Met exercise goal today _____

Days in a row of Lean Mode journaling _____    lbs.

Met food goal today _____

- free day _____

Glasses of water _____

# Lean Mode Food Diary **Daily Page** FOR _____ / _____ / _____

| What I ate/drank | Where/When | Quantity | Calories | Fat Grams | Carbs Grams | Fiber Grams | Protein Grams | |
|---|---|---|---|---|---|---|---|---|
| | | | | | | | | |
| | | | | | | | | |
| | | | | | | | | |
| | | | | | | | | |
| | | | | | | | | |
| | | | | | | | | |
| | | | | | | | | |
| | | | | | | | | |
| | | | | | | | | |
| | | | | | | | | |
| | | | | | | | | |
| | | | | | | | | |

**FOOD TOTALS:**

**Color in** the FoodDots above that show healthy eating.
Try to connect-the-FoodDots with color.

| | Where | When | Duration | Distance |
|---|---|---|---|---|
| Exercise | | | | |

**EXERCISE TOTALS:**

## Color in
today's PowerCircles!

Met exercise goal today _____

Days in a row of
Lean Mode journaling _____   lbs.

Met food goal today _____

- free day _____

Glasses of water _____

Su  M  Tu  W  Th  F  Sa   Select Day of Week

# Lean Mode Food Diary **Daily Page** FOR _____ / _____ / _____

| | What I ate/drank | Where/When | Quantity | Calories | Fat Grams | Carbs Grams | Fiber Grams | Protein Grams | |
|---|---|---|---|---|---|---|---|---|---|
| | | | | | | | | | |
| | | | | | | | | | |
| | | | | | | | | | |
| | | | | | | | | | |
| | | | | | | | | | |
| | | | | | | | | | |
| | | | | | | | | | |
| | | | | | | | | | |
| | | | | | | | | | |
| | | | | | | | | | |
| | | | | | | | | | |
| | | | | | | | | | |
| | | | | | | | | | |
| | | | | | | | | | |
| | | | | | | | | | |
| | **FOOD TOTALS:** | | | | | | | | |

**Color in** the FoodDots above that show healthy eating.
Try to connect-the-FoodDots with color.

| | Where | When | Duration | Distance |
|---|---|---|---|---|
| Exercise | | | | |
| | | | | |
| **EXERCISE TOTALS:** | | | | |

## Color in
today's PowerCircles!

Met exercise goal today _____

Days in a row of
Lean Mode journaling _____

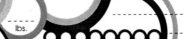  lbs.

Met food goal today _____

- free day _____

Glasses of water _____

# Complete Your **4Week Bubble**

Look back over your Weekly Tabs for the past 4 weeks and tally the results.

**4WEEK BUBBLE RECAP:** ___/___/___ thru ___/___/___

| | Start | End | + or − |
|---|---|---|---|
| Weight | | | |
| | | | |
| | | | |

**Yay!** I journaled every day

I journaled _____ days this period,
_____ days in a row this period,
and _____ days in a row to date.

The **REWARD** I gave myself for meeting all my weekly goals this period was:

_____
(Color in your **4WEEK BUBBLE** at right)

○ NO, I didn't meet all my weekly goals, but here's what I need to change to succeed next month:

_____
_____

**YES,** I met ALL my weekly goals!

---

Set up your Goals and Color Code for the WEEK of ___/___/___ thru ___/___/___   Journaling Week # _____

| **DAILY GOALS** (Your choice of sections below)<br>○ Same as last week | **WEEKLY GOALS**<br>○ Same as last week | **WEEKLY TAB**<br>Review your PowerCircles at week's end |
|---|---|---|
| **My daily food goal is:** _____ **calories**<br><br>My color for meeting all my daily food goals:<br>( )<br>( )<br>( )<br>( ) | I'll meet the goal at left at least _____ times per week | Did I meet my weekly goal at left?<br>**YES,** I met my weekly goal!<br>(Color it in) |
| **I'll include these healthy foods each day:**<br>FoodDot Color   Food Group/Item   Amount<br><br>Optional Lean Mode Life Day | I'll meet the goal at left at least<br><br>_____ times per week<br>_____ times per week<br>_____ times per week | Did I meet my weekly goal at left?<br>**YES,** I met my weekly goal!<br>(Color it in) |
| **I'll color in a** _____ **- free day**<br>(e.g. sugar-free, pastry-free, soda-free, etc.)<br><br>in this color in this spot in my PowerCircles: | I'll meet the goal at left at least _____ times per week | Did I meet my weekly goal at left?<br>**YES,** I met my weekly goal!<br>(Color it in) |
| **My daily exercise goal is:** _____<br><br>My color for meeting my daily exercise goal is: | I'll meet the goal at left at least _____ times per week | Did I meet my weekly goal at left?<br>**YES,** I met my weekly goal!<br>(Color it in) |

My **4WEEK BUBBLE REWARD** for meeting all my weekly goals will be: _____

Su M Tu W Th F Sa Select Day of Week

# Lean Mode Food Diary **Daily Page** FOR ____ / ____ / ____

| What I ate/drank | Where/When | Quantity | Calories | Fat Grams | Carbs Grams | Fiber Grams | Protein Grams | |
|---|---|---|---|---|---|---|---|---|
| | | | | | | | | |
| | | | | | | | | |
| | | | | | | | | |
| | | | | | | | | |
| | | | | | | | | |
| | | | | | | | | |
| | | | | | | | | |
| | | | | | | | | |
| | | | | | | | | |
| | | | | | | | | |
| | | | | | | | | |
| | | | | | | | | |
| | | | | | | | | |
| | | | | | | | | |
| | | | | | | | | |
| | | | | | | | | |
| | | | | | | | | |
| **FOOD TOTALS:** | | | | | | | | |

**Color in** the FoodDots above that show healthy eating.
Try to connect-the-FoodDots with color.

| | Where | When | Duration | Distance | |
|---|---|---|---|---|---|
| Exercise | | | | | |
| | | | | | |
| **EXERCISE TOTALS:** | | | | | |

## Color in today's PowerCircles!

Met exercise goal today ____

Days in a row of Lean Mode journaling ____

____ lbs.

Met food goal today ____

- free day ____

Glasses of water ____

# Lean Mode Food Diary **Daily Page** FOR ____ / ____ / ____

| What I ate/drank | Where/When | Quantity | Calories | Fat Grams | Carbs Grams | Fiber Grams | Protein Grams |
|---|---|---|---|---|---|---|---|
| | | | | | | | |
| | | | | | | | |
| | | | | | | | |
| | | | | | | | |
| | | | | | | | |
| | | | | | | | |
| | | | | | | | |
| | | | | | | | |
| | | | | | | | |
| | | | | | | | |
| | | | | | | | |
| | | | | | | | |
| | | | | | | | |
| **FOOD TOTALS:** | | | | | | | |

**Color in** the FoodDots above that show healthy eating.
Try to connect-the-FoodDots with color.

| | Where | When | Duration | Distance |
|---|---|---|---|---|
| Exercise | | | | |
| **EXERCISE TOTALS:** | | | | |

## Color in today's PowerCircles!

Met exercise goal today _____

Days in a row of
Lean Mode journaling

_____ lbs.

Met food goal today _____

- free day _____

Glasses of water _____

# Lean Mode Food Diary **Daily Page** FOR ___ / ___ / ___

| What I ate/drank | Where/When | Quantity | Calories | Fat Grams | Carbs Grams | Fiber Grams | Protein Grams |
|---|---|---|---|---|---|---|---|
| | | | | | | | |
| | | | | | | | |
| | | | | | | | |
| | | | | | | | |
| | | | | | | | |
| | | | | | | | |
| | | | | | | | |
| | | | | | | | |
| | | | | | | | |
| | | | | | | | |
| | | | | | | | |
| | | | | | | | |
| | | | | | | | |
| | | | | | | | |
| | | | | | | | |
| **FOOD TOTALS:** | | | | | | | |

**Color in** the FoodDots above that show healthy eating.
Try to connect-the-FoodDots with color.

| | Where | When | Duration | Distance |
|---|---|---|---|---|
| Exercise | | | | |
| **EXERCISE TOTALS:** | | | | |

## Color in today's PowerCircles!

Met exercise goal today _____

Met food goal today _____

Days in a row of Lean Mode journaling _____

___ lbs.

- free day _____

Glasses of water _____

(Su) (M) (Tu) (W) (Th) (F) (Sa)  **Select Day of Week**

# Lean Mode Food Diary **Daily Page** FOR ___ / ___ / ___

| What I ate/drank | Where/When | Quantity | Calories | Fat Grams | Carbs Grams | Fiber Grams | Protein Grams |
|---|---|---|---|---|---|---|---|
| | | | | | | | |
| | | | | | | | |
| | | | | | | | |
| | | | | | | | |
| | | | | | | | |
| | | | | | | | |
| | | | | | | | |
| | | | | | | | |
| | | | | | | | |
| | | | | | | | |
| | | | | | | | |
| | | | | | | | |
| | | | | | | | |
| | | | | | | | |
| | | | | | | | |
| | | | | | | | |
| **FOOD TOTALS:** | | | | | | | |

**Color in** the FoodDots above that show healthy eating.
Try to connect-the-FoodDots with color.

| | Where | When | Duration | Distance |
|---|---|---|---|---|
| Exercise | | | | |
| **EXERCISE TOTALS:** | | | | |

## Color in today's PowerCircles!

Met exercise goal today _____

Days in a row of Lean Mode journaling _____

_____ lbs.

Met food goal today _____

- free day _____

Glasses of water _____

# Lean Mode Food Diary **Daily Page** FOR _____ / ___ / _____

| What I ate/drank | Where/When | Quantity | Calories | Fat Grams | Carbs Grams | Fiber Grams | Protein Grams | |
|---|---|---|---|---|---|---|---|---|
| | | | | | | | | |
| | | | | | | | | |
| | | | | | | | | |
| | | | | | | | | |
| | | | | | | | | |
| | | | | | | | | |
| | | | | | | | | |
| | | | | | | | | |
| | | | | | | | | |
| | | | | | | | | |
| | | | | | | | | |
| | | | | | | | | |
| | | | | | | | | |
| | | | | | | | | |
| **FOOD TOTALS:** | | | | | | | | |

**Color in** the FoodDots above that show healthy eating. Try to connect-the-FoodDots with color.

| | Where | When | Duration | Distance | | |
|---|---|---|---|---|---|---|
| Exercise | | | | | | |
| **EXERCISE TOTALS:** | | | | | | |

## Color in today's PowerCircles!

Met exercise goal today _____

Days in a row of Lean Mode journaling _____

lbs.

Met food goal today _____

- free day _____

Glasses of water _____

# Lean Mode Food Diary **Daily Page** FOR ___ / ___ / ___

| What I ate/drank | Where/When | Quantity | Calories | Fat Grams | Carbs Grams | Fiber Grams | Protein Grams |
|---|---|---|---|---|---|---|---|
| | | | | | | | |
| | | | | | | | |
| | | | | | | | |
| | | | | | | | |
| | | | | | | | |
| | | | | | | | |
| | | | | | | | |
| | | | | | | | |
| | | | | | | | |
| | | | | | | | |
| | | | | | | | |
| | | | | | | | |
| **FOOD TOTALS:** | | | | | | | |

**Color in** the FoodDots above that show healthy eating.
Try to connect-the-FoodDots with color.

| | Where | When | Duration | Distance |
|---|---|---|---|---|
| Exercise | | | | |
| **EXERCISE TOTALS:** | | | | |

## Color in today's PowerCircles!

Met exercise goal today ___

Met food goal today ___

Days in a row of Lean Mode journaling ___

___ lbs.

___ - free day

Glasses of water ___

Su M Tu W Th F Sa Select Day of Week

# Lean Mode Food Diary **Daily Page** FOR _____ / _____ / _____

| | What I ate/drank | Where/When | Quantity | Calories | Fat Grams | Carbs Grams | Fiber Grams | Protein Grams | |
|---|---|---|---|---|---|---|---|---|---|
| | | | | | | | | | |
| | | | | | | | | | |
| | | | | | | | | | |
| | | | | | | | | | |
| | | | | | | | | | |
| | | | | | | | | | |
| | | | | | | | | | |
| | | | | | | | | | |
| | | | | | | | | | |
| | | | | | | | | | |
| | | | | | | | | | |
| | | | | | | | | | |
| **FOOD TOTALS:** | | | | | | | | | |

**Color in** the FoodDots above that show healthy eating.
Try to connect-the-FoodDots with color.

| | Where | When | Duration | Distance | |
|---|---|---|---|---|---|
| Exercise | | | | | |
| **EXERCISE TOTALS:** | | | | | |

## Color in
today's PowerCircles!

Met exercise goal today _____

Met food goal today _____

Days in a row of
Lean Mode journaling _____

lbs.

- free day _____

Glasses of water _____

# Fill in Your **Color Code & Goals Page**

Take baby steps! Gradually build better habits by setting realistic goals here.

**NOTES:**

Set up your Goals and Color Code for the WEEK of _ _ _ _/_ _ _ _/_ _ _ _ thru _ _ _ _/_ _ _ _/_ _ _ _   Journaling Week # _ _ _ _ _ _

| **DAILY GOALS** (Your choice of sections below) ○ Same as last week | **WEEKLY GOALS** ○ Same as last week | **WEEKLY TAB** Review your PowerCircles at week's end |
|---|---|---|
| **My daily food goal is:** ........... **calories** <br> My color for meeting all <br> my daily food goals: <br> ( ) <br> ( ) <br> ( ) <br> ( ) | I'll meet the goal at left at least ......... times per week | Did I meet my weekly goal at left? **YES, I met my weekly goal!** (Color it in) |
| **I'll include these healthy foods each day:** <br> FoodDot Color    Food Group/Item    Amount <br> _Optional Lean Mode Lite Day_ | I'll meet the goal at left at least <br> ........ times per week <br> ........ times per week <br> ........ times per week | Did I meet my weekly goal at left? **YES, I met my weekly goal!** (Color it in) |
| **I'll color in a** _____ **- free day** <br> (e.g. sugar-free, pastry-free, soda-free, etc.) <br> in this color in this spot in <br> my PowerCircles: | I'll meet the goal at left at least ......... times per week | Did I meet my weekly goal at left? **YES, I met my weekly goal!** (Color it in) |
| **My daily exercise goal is:** <br> My color for meeting my <br> daily exercise goal is: | I'll meet the goal at left at least ......... times per week | Did I meet my weekly goal at left? **YES, I met my weekly goal!** (Color it in) |

My **4WEEK BUBBLE REWARD** for meeting all my weekly goals will be: _____

Su  M  Tu  W  Th  F  Sa    Select Day of Week

# Lean Mode Food Diary **Daily Page** FOR _____ / _____ / _____

| What I ate/drank | Where/When | Quantity | Calories | Fat Grams | Carbs Grams | Fiber Grams | Protein Grams |
|---|---|---|---|---|---|---|---|
| | | | | | | | |
| | | | | | | | |
| | | | | | | | |
| | | | | | | | |
| | | | | | | | |
| | | | | | | | |
| | | | | | | | |
| | | | | | | | |
| | | | | | | | |
| | | | | | | | |
| | | | | | | | |
| | | | | | | | |
| **FOOD TOTALS:** | | | | | | | |

**Color in** the FoodDots above that show healthy eating.
Try to connect-the-FoodDots with color.

| | Where | When | Duration | Distance |
|---|---|---|---|---|
| Exercise | | | | |
| **EXERCISE TOTALS:** | | | | |

## Color in today's PowerCircles!

Met exercise goal today _____

Days in a row of Lean Mode journaling _____

_____ lbs.

Met food goal today _____

_____ - free day

Glasses of water _____

# Lean Mode Food Diary **Daily Page** FOR ___/___/___

| | What I ate/drank | Where/When | Quantity | Calories | Fat Grams | Carbs Grams | Fiber Grams | Protein Grams |
|---|---|---|---|---|---|---|---|---|
| | | | | | | | | |
| | | | | | | | | |
| | | | | | | | | |
| | | | | | | | | |
| | | | | | | | | |
| | | | | | | | | |
| | | | | | | | | |
| | | | | | | | | |
| | | | | | | | | |
| | | | | | | | | |
| | | | | | | | | |
| | | | | | | | | |
| | | | | | | | | |
| | FOOD TOTALS: | | | | | | | |

**Color in** the FoodDots above that show healthy eating.
Try to connect-the-FoodDots with color.

| | Where | When | Duration | Distance |
|---|---|---|---|---|
| Exercise | | | | |
| | | | | |
| EXERCISE TOTALS: | | | | |

## Color in
## today's PowerCircles!

Met exercise goal today _____

Met food goal today _____

\- free day _____

Days in a row of
Lean Mode journaling _____

lbs.

Glasses of water _____

# Lean Mode Food Diary **Daily Page** FOR ____ / ____ / ____

| What I ate/drank | Where/When | Quantity | Calories | Fat Grams | Carbs Grams | Fiber Grams | Protein Grams | |
|---|---|---|---|---|---|---|---|---|
| | | | | | | | | |
| | | | | | | | | |
| | | | | | | | | |
| | | | | | | | | |
| | | | | | | | | |
| | | | | | | | | |
| | | | | | | | | |
| | | | | | | | | |
| | | | | | | | | |
| | | | | | | | | |
| | | | | | | | | |
| | | | | | | | | |
| | | | | | | | | |
| **FOOD TOTALS:** | | | | | | | | |

**Color in** the FoodDots above that show healthy eating.
Try to connect-the-FoodDots with color.

| | Where | When | Duration | Distance | |
|---|---|---|---|---|---|
| Exercise | | | | | |
| **EXERCISE TOTALS:** | | | | | |

## Color in today's PowerCircles!

Met exercise goal today _____

Met food goal today _____

- free day

Days in a row of Lean Mode journaling _____     lbs.

Glasses of water _____

# Lean Mode Food Diary **Daily Page** FOR ____ / ____ / ____

| | What I ate/drank | Where/When | Quantity | Calories | Fat Grams | Carbs Grams | Fiber Grams | Protein Grams |
|---|---|---|---|---|---|---|---|---|
| | | | | | | | | |
| | | | | | | | | |
| | | | | | | | | |
| | | | | | | | | |
| | | | | | | | | |
| | | | | | | | | |
| | | | | | | | | |
| | | | | | | | | |
| | | | | | | | | |
| | | | | | | | | |
| | | | | | | | | |
| | | | | | | | | |
| | | | | | | | | |
| | | | | | | | | |
| | | | | | | | | |
| | | | | | | | | |
| | | **FOOD TOTALS:** | | | | | | |

**Color in** the FoodDots above that show healthy eating.
Try to connect-the-FoodDots with color.

| | Where | When | Duration | Distance | |
|---|---|---|---|---|---|
| Exercise | | | | | |
| | **EXERCISE TOTALS:** | | | | |

## Color in today's PowerCircles!

Met exercise goal today ____

Days in a row of Lean Mode journaling ____

lbs.

Met food goal today ____

- free day ____

Glasses of water ____

Su  M  Tu  W  Th  F  Sa    Select Day of Week

# Lean Mode Food Diary **Daily Page**  FOR  _____ / _____ / _____

| What I ate/drank | Where/When | Quantity | Calories | Fat Grams | Carbs Grams | Fiber Grams | Protein Grams |
|---|---|---|---|---|---|---|---|
| | | | | | | | |
| | | | | | | | |
| | | | | | | | |
| | | | | | | | |
| | | | | | | | |
| | | | | | | | |
| | | | | | | | |
| | | | | | | | |
| | | | | | | | |
| | | | | | | | |
| | | | | | | | |
| | | | | | | | |
| | | | | | | | |
| | | | | | | | |
| **FOOD TOTALS:** | | | | | | | |

**Color in** the FoodDots above that show healthy eating.
Try to connect-the-FoodDots with color.

| | Where | When | Duration | Distance |
|---|---|---|---|---|
| Exercise | | | | |
| **EXERCISE TOTALS:** | | | | |

## Color in
### today's PowerCircles!

Met exercise goal today _____

Days in a row of
Lean Mode journaling _____        lbs.

Met food goal today _____

_____ - free day

Glasses of water _____

# Lean Mode Food Diary **Daily Page** FOR ___ / ___ / ___

| What I ate/drank | Where/When | Quantity | Calories | Fat Grams | Carbs Grams | Fiber Grams | Protein Grams |
|---|---|---|---|---|---|---|---|
| | | | | | | | |
| | | | | | | | |
| | | | | | | | |
| | | | | | | | |
| | | | | | | | |
| | | | | | | | |
| | | | | | | | |
| | | | | | | | |
| | | | | | | | |
| | | | | | | | |
| | | | | | | | |
| | | | | | | | |
| | | | | | | | |
| | | | | | | | |
| | | | | | | | |
| **FOOD TOTALS:** | | | | | | | |

**Color in** the FoodDots above that show healthy eating.
Try to connect-the-FoodDots with color.

| | Where | When | Duration | Distance |
|---|---|---|---|---|
| Exercise | | | | |
| | | | | |
| **EXERCISE TOTALS:** | | | | |

## Color in today's PowerCircles!

Met exercise goal today ___

Days in a row of Lean Mode journaling ___

___ lbs.

Met food goal today ___

- free day ___

Glasses of water ___

# Lean Mode Food Diary **Daily Page** FOR _____/_____/_____

| What I ate/drank | Where/When | Quantity | Calories | Fat Grams | Carbs Grams | Fiber Grams | Protein Grams |
|---|---|---|---|---|---|---|---|
|  |  |  |  |  |  |  |  |
|  |  |  |  |  |  |  |  |
|  |  |  |  |  |  |  |  |
|  |  |  |  |  |  |  |  |
|  |  |  |  |  |  |  |  |
|  |  |  |  |  |  |  |  |
|  |  |  |  |  |  |  |  |
|  |  |  |  |  |  |  |  |
|  |  |  |  |  |  |  |  |
|  |  |  |  |  |  |  |  |
|  |  |  |  |  |  |  |  |
|  |  |  |  |  |  |  |  |
|  |  |  |  |  |  |  |  |
| **FOOD TOTALS:** |  |  |  |  |  |  |  |

**Color in** the FoodDots above that show healthy eating.
Try to connect-the-FoodDots with color.

| Exercise | Where | When | Duration | Distance |
|---|---|---|---|---|
|  |  |  |  |  |
|  |  |  |  |  |
| **EXERCISE TOTALS:** |  |  |  |  |

# Color in
## today's PowerCircles!

Met exercise goal today _____

Days in a row of
Lean Mode journaling _____

_____ Met food goal today

_____ - free day

lbs.   _____ Glasses of water

# Fill in Your **Color Code & Goals Page**

Take baby steps! Gradually build better habits by setting realistic goals here.

**NOTES:**

Set up your Goals and Color Code for the WEEK of ___/___/____ thru ____/___/____   Journaling Week # _____

| **DAILY GOALS** (Your choice of sections below)<br>◯ Same as last week | **WEEKLY GOALS**<br>◯ Same as last week | **WEEKLY TAB**<br>Review your PowerCircles at week's end |
|---|---|---|
| **My daily food goal is:** _____ **calories**<br><br>My color for meeting all<br>my daily food goals:<br>( )  ( )  ( )  ( ) | I'll meet the goal at left<br>at least _____ times<br>per week | Did I meet my weekly goal at left?  **YES, I met my weekly goal!**<br>(Color it in) |
| **I'll include these healthy foods each day:**<br>FoodDot Color     Food Group/Item     Amount<br><br>Optional Lean Mode Life Day | I'll meet the goal at left<br>at least<br><br>_____ times per week<br>_____ times per week<br>_____ times per week | Did I meet my weekly goal at left?  **YES, I met my weekly goal!**<br>(Color it in) |
| **I'll color in a** _____ **- free day**<br>(e.g. sugar-free, pastry-free, soda-free, etc.)<br><br>in this color in this spot in<br>my PowerCircles: | I'll meet the goal at left<br>at least _____ times<br>per week | Did I meet my weekly goal at left?  **YES, I met my weekly goal!**<br>(Color it in) |
| **My daily exercise goal is:** _____<br><br>My color for meeting my<br>daily exercise goal is: | I'll meet the goal at left<br>at least _____ times<br>per week | Did I meet my weekly goal at left?  **YES, I met my weekly goal!**<br>(Color it in) |

My **4WEEK BUBBLE REWARD** for meeting all my weekly goals will be: _____

Su  M  Tu  W  Th  F  Sa   Select Day of Week

# Lean Mode Food Diary **Daily Page** FOR _____ / ____ / _____

| | What I ate/drank | Where/When | Quantity | Calories | Fat Grams | Carbs Grams | Fiber Grams | Protein Grams | |
|---|---|---|---|---|---|---|---|---|---|
| | | | | | | | | | |

**FOOD TOTALS:**

**Color in** the FoodDots above that show healthy eating.
Try to connect-the-FoodDots with color.

| | Where | When | Duration | Distance | |
|---|---|---|---|---|---|
| Exercise | | | | | |

**EXERCISE TOTALS:**

## Color in today's PowerCircles!

Met exercise goal today

Days in a row of Lean Mode journaling

lbs.

Met food goal today

- free day

Glasses of water

# Lean Mode Food Diary **Daily Page** FOR ___ / ___ / ___

| | What I ate/drank | Where/When | Quantity | Calories | Fat Grams | Carbs Grams | Fiber Grams | Protein Grams |
|---|---|---|---|---|---|---|---|---|
| | | | | | | | | |
| | | | | | | | | |
| | | | | | | | | |
| | | | | | | | | |
| | | | | | | | | |
| | | | | | | | | |
| | | | | | | | | |
| | | | | | | | | |
| | | | | | | | | |
| | | | | | | | | |
| | | | | | | | | |
| | | | | | | | | |
| | | | | | | | | |
| | | | | | | | | |
| | | | | | | | | |

**FOOD TOTALS:**

**Color in** the FoodDots above that show healthy eating.
Try to connect-the-FoodDots with color.

| | Where | When | Duration | Distance | |
|---|---|---|---|---|---|
| Exercise | | | | | |

**EXERCISE TOTALS:**

# Color in
## today's PowerCircles!

Met exercise goal today ___                                           Met food goal today ___

                                                                      - free day ___

Days in a row of
Lean Mode journaling ___           ___ lbs.              Glasses of water ___

Su  M  Tu  W  Th  F  Sa    Select Day
of Week

# Lean Mode Food Diary **Daily Page**  FOR _____ / ____ / _____

| What I ate/drank | Where/When | Quantity | Calories | Fat Grams | Carbs Grams | Fiber Grams | Protein Grams |
|---|---|---|---|---|---|---|---|
|  |  |  |  |  |  |  |  |
|  |  |  |  |  |  |  |  |
|  |  |  |  |  |  |  |  |
|  |  |  |  |  |  |  |  |
|  |  |  |  |  |  |  |  |
|  |  |  |  |  |  |  |  |
|  |  |  |  |  |  |  |  |
|  |  |  |  |  |  |  |  |
|  |  |  |  |  |  |  |  |
|  |  |  |  |  |  |  |  |
|  |  |  |  |  |  |  |  |
|  |  |  |  |  |  |  |  |
|  |  |  |  |  |  |  |  |

**FOOD TOTALS:**

**Color in** the FoodDots above that show healthy eating.
Try to connect-the-FoodDots with color.

|  | Where | When | Duration | Distance |
|---|---|---|---|---|
| Exercise |  |  |  |  |

**EXERCISE TOTALS:**

## Color in
today's PowerCircles!

Met exercise goal today _____

Met food goal today _____

- free day _____

Days in a row of
Lean Mode journaling _____

_____ lbs.

Glasses of water _____

Su M Tu W Th F Sa  **Select Day of Week**

# Lean Mode Food Diary **Daily Page** FOR ___ / ___ / ___

| What I ate/drank | Where/When | Quantity | Calories | Fat Grams | Carbs Grams | Fiber Grams | Protein Grams |
|---|---|---|---|---|---|---|---|
| | | | | | | | |
| | | | | | | | |
| | | | | | | | |
| | | | | | | | |
| | | | | | | | |
| | | | | | | | |
| | | | | | | | |
| | | | | | | | |
| | | | | | | | |
| | | | | | | | |
| | | | | | | | |
| | | | | | | | |
| | | | | | | | |
| | | | | | | | |
| **FOOD TOTALS:** | | | | | | | |

**Color in** the FoodDots above that show healthy eating.
Try to connect-the-FoodDots with color.

| | Where | When | Duration | Distance |
|---|---|---|---|---|
| Exercise | | | | |
| **EXERCISE TOTALS:** | | | | |

## Color in
### today's PowerCircles!

Met exercise goal today _____

Days in a row of
Lean Mode journaling _____

lbs.

Met food goal today _____

- free day _____

Glasses of water _____

Su M Tu W Th F Sa  Select Day of Week

# Lean Mode Food Diary **Daily Page** FOR ___ / ___ / ___

| What I ate/drank | Where/When | Quantity | Calories | Fat Grams | Carbs Grams | Fiber Grams | Protein Grams | |
|---|---|---|---|---|---|---|---|---|
| | | | | | | | | |
| | | | | | | | | |
| | | | | | | | | |
| | | | | | | | | |
| | | | | | | | | |
| | | | | | | | | |
| | | | | | | | | |
| | | | | | | | | |
| | | | | | | | | |
| | | | | | | | | |
| | | | | | | | | |
| | | | | | | | | |
| | | | | | | | | |
| **FOOD TOTALS:** | | | | | | | | |

**Color in** the FoodDots above that show healthy eating.
Try to connect-the-FoodDots with color.

| | Where | When | Duration | Distance | |
|---|---|---|---|---|---|
| Exercise | | | | | |
| **EXERCISE TOTALS:** | | | | | |

# Color in today's PowerCircles!

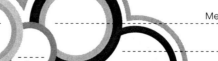

Met exercise goal today ___

Days in a row of Lean Mode journaling ___

___ lbs.

Met food goal today ___

- free day ___

Glasses of water ___

# Lean Mode Food Diary **Daily Page** FOR _____ / _____ / _____

| | What I ate/drank | Where/When | Quantity | Calories | Fat Grams | Carbs Grams | Fiber Grams | Protein Grams |
|---|---|---|---|---|---|---|---|---|
| | | | | | | | | |
| | | | | | | | | |
| | | | | | | | | |
| | | | | | | | | |
| | | | | | | | | |
| | | | | | | | | |
| | | | | | | | | |
| | | | | | | | | |
| | | | | | | | | |
| | | | | | | | | |
| | | | | | | | | |
| | | | | | | | | |
| | | | | | | | | |
| | **FOOD TOTALS:** | | | | | | | |

**Color in** the FoodDots above that show healthy eating.
Try to connect-the-FoodDots with color.

| | | Where | When | Duration | Distance |
|---|---|---|---|---|---|
| Exercise | | | | | |
| | **EXERCISE TOTALS:** | | | | |

## Color in today's PowerCircles!

Met exercise goal today _____

Met food goal today _____

Days in a row of Lean Mode journaling _____

_____ lbs.

_____ - free day

Glasses of water _____

Su  M  Tu  W  Th  F  Sa    Select Day of Week

# Lean Mode Food Diary **Daily Page** FOR _____ / _____ / _____

| What I ate/drank | Where/When | Quantity | Calories | Fat Grams | Carbs Grams | Fiber Grams | Protein Grams | |
|---|---|---|---|---|---|---|---|---|
| | | | | | | | | |
| | | | | | | | | |
| | | | | | | | | |
| | | | | | | | | |
| | | | | | | | | |
| | | | | | | | | |
| | | | | | | | | |
| | | | | | | | | |
| | | | | | | | | |
| | | | | | | | | |
| | | | | | | | | |
| | | | | | | | | |

**FOOD TOTALS:**

**Color in** the FoodDots above that show healthy eating.
Try to connect-the-FoodDots with color.

| | Where | When | Duration | Distance | |
|---|---|---|---|---|---|
| Exercise | | | | | |

**EXERCISE TOTALS:**

## Color in today's PowerCircles!

Met exercise goal today _____

Met food goal today _____

- free day _____

Days in a row of Lean Mode journaling _____

lbs.

Glasses of water _____

# Fill in Your **Color Code & Goals Page**

Take baby steps! Gradually build better habits by setting realistic goals here.

**NOTES:**

Set up your Goals and Color Code for the WEEK of _ _ _ _ / _ _ _ / _ _ _ _ thru _ _ _ _ / _ _ _ / _ _ _ _ Journaling Week # _ _ _ _ _ _

| **DAILY GOALS** (Your choice of sections below)<br>○ Same as last week | **WEEKLY GOALS**<br>○ Same as last week | **WEEKLY TAB**<br>Review your PowerCircles at week's end |
|---|---|---|
| **My daily food goal is:** _____ **calories**<br><br>My color for meeting all<br>my daily food goals:<br>(   )<br>(   )<br>(   )<br>(   ) | I'll meet the goal at left<br>at least _____ times<br>per week | Did I meet my weekly goal at left?<br>**YES,** I met my weekly goal!<br>(Color it in) |
| **I'll include these healthy foods each day:**<br>FoodDot Color    Food Group/Item    Amount<br><br>Optional Lean Mode Lite Day | I'll meet the goal at left<br>at least<br><br>_____ times per week<br>_____ times per week<br>_____ times per week | Did I meet my weekly goal at left?<br>**YES,** I met my weekly goal!<br>(Color it in) |
| **I'll color in a** _____ **- free day**<br>(e.g. sugar-free, pastry-free, soda-free, etc.)<br><br>in this color in this spot in<br>my PowerCircles: | I'll meet the goal at left<br>at least _____ times<br>per week | Did I meet my weekly goal at left?<br>**YES,** I met my weekly goal!<br>(Color it in) |
| **My daily exercise goal is:** _____<br><br>My color for meeting my<br>daily exercise goal is: | I'll meet the goal at left<br>at least _____ times<br>per week | Did I meet my weekly goal at left?<br>**YES,** I met my weekly goal!<br>(Color it in) |

My **4WEEK BUBBLE REWARD** for meeting all my weekly goals will be: _____

Su M Tu W Th F Sa  Select Day of Week

# Lean Mode Food Diary **Daily Page** FOR _____ / _____ / _____

| | What I ate/drank | Where/When | Quantity | Calories | Fat Grams | Carbs Grams | Fiber Grams | Protein Grams | |
|---|---|---|---|---|---|---|---|---|---|
| | | | | | | | | | |
| | | | | | | | | | |
| | | | | | | | | | |
| | | | | | | | | | |
| | | | | | | | | | |
| | | | | | | | | | |
| | | | | | | | | | |
| | | | | | | | | | |
| | | | | | | | | | |
| | | | | | | | | | |
| | | | | | | | | | |
| | | | | | | | | | |
| | | | | | | | | | |
| | | **FOOD TOTALS:** | | | | | | | |

**Color in** the FoodDots above that show healthy eating.
Try to connect-the-FoodDots with color.

| | Where | When | Duration | Distance | | |
|---|---|---|---|---|---|---|
| Exercise | | | | | | |
| | **EXERCISE TOTALS:** | | | | | |

## Color in today's PowerCircles!

Met exercise goal today _____

Met food goal today _____

- free day

Days in a row of Lean Mode journaling _____

lbs.

Glasses of water

(Su) (M) (Tu) (W) (Th) (F) (Sa)  Select Day
of Week

# Lean Mode Food Diary **Daily Page**  FOR  _____ / _____ / _____

| | What I ate/drank | Where/When | Quantity | Calories | Fat Grams | Carbs Grams | Fiber Grams | Protein Grams |
|---|---|---|---|---|---|---|---|---|
| | | | | | | | | |
| | | | | | | | | |
| | | | | | | | | |
| | | | | | | | | |
| | | | | | | | | |
| | | | | | | | | |
| | | | | | | | | |
| | | | | | | | | |
| | | | | | | | | |
| | | | | | | | | |
| | | | | | | | | |
| | | | | | | | | |
| | | | | | | | | |
| | | | | | | | | |
| | | | | | | | | |

**FOOD TOTALS:**

**Color in** the FoodDots above that show healthy eating.
Try to connect-the-FoodDots with color.

| | Where | When | Duration | Distance |
|---|---|---|---|---|
| Exercise | | | | |

**EXERCISE TOTALS:**

## Color in
today's PowerCircles!

Met exercise goal today _____

Days in a row of
Lean Mode journaling _____          lbs.

Met food goal today _____

- free day _____

Glasses of water _____

# Lean Mode Food Diary **Daily Page** FOR ___/___/___

| What I ate/drank | Where/When | Quantity | Calories | Fat Grams | Carbs Grams | Fiber Grams | Protein Grams | |
|---|---|---|---|---|---|---|---|---|
| | | | | | | | | |
| | | | | | | | | |
| | | | | | | | | |
| | | | | | | | | |
| | | | | | | | | |
| | | | | | | | | |
| | | | | | | | | |
| | | | | | | | | |
| | | | | | | | | |
| | | | | | | | | |
| | | | | | | | | |
| **FOOD TOTALS:** | | | | | | | | |

**Color in** the FoodDots above that show healthy eating.
Try to connect-the-FoodDots with color.

| | Where | When | Duration | Distance | |
|---|---|---|---|---|---|
| Exercise | | | | | |
| **EXERCISE TOTALS:** | | | | | |

## Color in today's PowerCircles!

Met exercise goal today ......................................

Days in a row of Lean Mode journaling ..................

lbs.

Met food goal today ......................................

- free day

Glasses of water

(Su) (M) (Tu) (W) (Th) (F) (Sa)  Select Day of Week

# Lean Mode Food Diary **Daily Page** FOR _____ / _____ / _____

| What I ate/drank | Where/When | Quantity | Calories | Fat Grams | Carbs Grams | Fiber Grams | Protein Grams |
|---|---|---|---|---|---|---|---|
| | | | | | | | |
| | | | | | | | |
| | | | | | | | |
| | | | | | | | |
| | | | | | | | |
| | | | | | | | |
| | | | | | | | |
| | | | | | | | |
| | | | | | | | |
| | | | | | | | |
| | | | | | | | |
| | | | | | | | |
| | | | | | | | |
| | | | | | | | |
| **FOOD TOTALS:** | | | | | | | |

**Color in** the FoodDots above that show healthy eating.
Try to connect-the-FoodDots with color.

| | Where | When | Duration | Distance |
|---|---|---|---|---|
| Exercise | | | | |
| **EXERCISE TOTALS:** | | | | |

## Color in today's PowerCircles!

Met exercise goal today _____

Days in a row of Lean Mode journaling _____

_____ lbs.

Met food goal today _____

- free day _____

Glasses of water _____

(Su) (M) (Tu) (W) (Th) (F) (Sa)  Select Day of Week

# Lean Mode Food Diary **Daily Page**  FOR _____ / _____ / _____

| What I ate/drank | Where/When | Quantity | Calories | Fat Grams | Carbs Grams | Fiber Grams | Protein Grams |
|---|---|---|---|---|---|---|---|
| | | | | | | | |
| | | | | | | | |
| | | | | | | | |
| | | | | | | | |
| | | | | | | | |
| | | | | | | | |
| | | | | | | | |
| | | | | | | | |
| | | | | | | | |
| | | | | | | | |
| | | | | | | | |
| | | | | | | | |
| | | | | | | | |
| **FOOD TOTALS:** | | | | | | | |

**Color in** the FoodDots above that show healthy eating.
Try to connect-the-FoodDots with color.

| | Where | When | Duration | Distance |
|---|---|---|---|---|
| Exercise | | | | |
| **EXERCISE TOTALS:** | | | | |

## Color in
### today's PowerCircles!

Met exercise goal today ------------------------------

Days in a row of
Lean Mode journaling

lbs.

Met food goal today

- free day

Glasses of water

# Lean Mode Food Diary **Daily Page** FOR ___/___/___

| | What I ate/drank | Where/When | Quantity | Calories | Fat Grams | Carbs Grams | Fiber Grams | Protein Grams |
|---|---|---|---|---|---|---|---|---|
| | | | | | | | | |
| | | | | | | | | |
| | | | | | | | | |
| | | | | | | | | |
| | | | | | | | | |
| | | | | | | | | |
| | | | | | | | | |
| | | | | | | | | |
| | | | | | | | | |
| | | | | | | | | |
| | | | | | | | | |
| | | | | | | | | |
| | **FOOD TOTALS:** | | | | | | | |

**Color in** the FoodDots above that show healthy eating.
Try to connect-the-FoodDots with color.

| | Where | When | Duration | Distance |
|---|---|---|---|---|
| Exercise | | | | |
| **EXERCISE TOTALS:** | | | | |

# Color in
## today's PowerCircles!

Met exercise goal today ___

Days in a row of
Lean Mode journaling ___

lbs. ___

Met food goal today ___

- free day ___

Glasses of water ___

Su M Tu W Th F Sa   Select Day of Week

# Lean Mode Food Diary **Daily Page** FOR ___/___/___

| What I ate/drank | Where/When | Quantity | Calories | Fat Grams | Carbs Grams | Fiber Grams | Protein Grams | |
|---|---|---|---|---|---|---|---|---|
| | | | | | | | | |
| | | | | | | | | |
| | | | | | | | | |
| | | | | | | | | |
| | | | | | | | | |
| | | | | | | | | |
| | | | | | | | | |
| | | | | | | | | |
| | | | | | | | | |
| | | | | | | | | |
| | | | | | | | | |
| **FOOD TOTALS:** | | | | | | | | |

**Color in** the FoodDots above that show healthy eating.
Try to connect-the-FoodDots with color.

| | Where | When | Duration | Distance | |
|---|---|---|---|---|---|
| Exercise | | | | | |
| **EXERCISE TOTALS:** | | | | | |

## Color in today's PowerCircles!

Met exercise goal today ................................................. Met food goal today

.......................... - free day

Days in a row of
Lean Mode journaling ............... lbs. ............... Glasses of water

# Complete Your **4Week Bubble**

Look back over your Weekly Tabs for the past 4 weeks and tally the results.

**4WEEK BUBBLE RECAP:** ___/___/___ thru ___/___/___

| | Start | End | + or – |
|---|---|---|---|
| Weight | | | |
| | | | |
| | | | |

**Yay!** I journaled every day

I journaled _____ days this period,
_____ days in a row this period,
and _____ days in a row to date.

The **REWARD** I gave myself for meeting all my weekly goals this period was:

_____

(Color in your **4WEEK BUBBLE** at right)

○ NO, I didn't meet all my weekly goals, but here's what I need to change to succeed next month:

_____

**YES,** I met ALL my weekly goals!

Set up your Goals and Color Code for the WEEK of ___/___/___ thru ___/___/___    Journaling Week # _____

**DAILY GOALS** (Your choice of sections below)
○ Same as last week

**WEEKLY GOALS**
○ Same as last week

**WEEKLY TAB**
Review your PowerCircles at week's end

My daily food goal is: _____ calories

My color for meeting all my daily food goals:
_____ (   )
_____ (   )
_____ (   )
_____ (   )

I'll meet the goal at left at least _____ times per week

Did I meet my weekly goal at left?

**YES,** I met my weekly goal!

(Color it in)

I'll include these healthy foods each day:

FoodDot Color    Food Group/Item    Amount

I'll meet the goal at left at least

_____ times per week
_____ times per week
_____ times per week

Did I meet my weekly goal at left?

**YES,** I met my weekly goal!

(Color it in)

I'll color in a _____ - free day
(e.g. sugar-free, pastry-free, soda-free, etc.)

in this color in this spot in my PowerCircles:

I'll meet the goal at left at least _____ times per week

Did I meet my weekly goal at left?

**YES,** I met my weekly goal!

(Color it in)

My daily exercise goal is: _____

My color for meeting my daily exercise goal is:

I'll meet the goal at left at least _____ times per week

Did I meet my weekly goal at left?

**YES,** I met my weekly goal!

(Color it in)

**It's time to order a new Lean Mode, Color Code Food Diary!**    www.colorcodemode.com

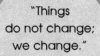

"Things
do not change;
we change."

*Henry David Thoreau*
*(1817 - 1862)*

# VI.   Your Half Year In Lean Mode

After 28 weeks of keeping your Lean Mode
Food Diary, rate your habits again at right,
then look back at how you rated them at
the beginning of Chapter III. Revisit your
Starting Stats and compare them to your
Half Year Stats.

What habit(s) have you changed the most?

What has been your biggest change or
accomplishment?

Do you feel more in control of your habits?

How have you surprised yourself?

How have you influenced others?

What was your best reward?

What's your next habit to target through
Lean Mode?

How would you rate your eating habits in terms of
controlling portion size and the overall amount of
food you eat each day?

I'm doing
everything
wrong
①  ②  ③  ④  ⑤  ⑥  ⑦  ⑧
I'm doing
everything
positive I can

Rate your eating habits in terms of the nutritional
value and soundness of the foods you eat.

①  ②  ③  ④  ⑤  ⑥  ⑦  ⑧

How many hours of low intensity exercise do you get,
on average, each week?

①  ②  ③  ④  ⑤  ⑥  ⑦  ⑧

How many hours of moderate (enough to break
a sweat) to high-intensity exercise do you get, on
average, each week?

①  ②  ③  ④  ⑤  ⑥  ⑦  ⑧

How many eight-ounce glasses of water do you
drink each day?

①  ②  ③  ④  ⑤  ⑥  ⑦  ⑧

## Your Half Year In Lean Mode

What was your favorite highlighter color to use?

- - - - - - - - - - - -

# Congratulations!

You've been in Lean Mode for 28 weeks (about a half year.) Look back over all your 4Week Bubble pages. Write in the start and end dates below, then color in the 4Week Bubbles where you met all your weekly goals.

- - /- - /- - -    - - /- - /- - -    - - /- - /- - -    - - /- - /- - -    - - /- - /- - -    - - /- - /- - -    - - /- - /- - -

**YES,** I met ALL my weekly goals!    **YES,** I met ALL my weekly goals!    **YES,** I met ALL my weekly goals!    **YES,** I met ALL my weekly goals!    **YES,** I met ALL my weekly goals!    **YES,** I met ALL my weekly goals!    **YES,** I met ALL my weekly goals!

- - /- - /- - -    - - /- - /- - -    - - /- - /- - -    - - /- - /- - -    - - /- - /- - -    - - /- - /- - -    - - /- - /- - -

Every bubble is an accomplishment.
Special congratulations if you can connect all seven!
What will be your extra-special reward for that?

_____

CHANGE YOUR HABITS—
CHANGE YOUR WORLD.

"We are what we repeatedly do. Excellence then, is not an act, but a habit."

*Aristotle (384-322 B.C.)*

What was your longest number of Lean Mode journaling days in a row? - - - - - - - -

Healthy habits continually evolve, so we hope you'll stay in Lean Mode for many years to come. You can track your Lean Mode Years here. Thanks, and we wish you a lifetime of non-stop great health!

Year 1    Year 2    Year 3    Year 4    Year 5    Year 6    Year 7    Year 8    Year 9    Year 10

www.colorcodemode.com

## october 2008

| S | M | T | W | T | F | S |
|---|---|---|---|---|---|---|
|   |   |   | 1 | 2 | 3 | 4 |
| 5 | 6 | 7 | 8 | 9 | 10 | 11 |
| 12 | 13 | 14 | 15 | 16 | 17 | 18 |
| 19 | 20 | 21 | 22 | 23 | 24 | 25 |
| 26 | 27 | 28 | 29 | 30 | 31 |   |

## november 2008

| S | M | T | W | T | F | S |
|---|---|---|---|---|---|---|
|   |   |   |   |   |   | 1 |
| 2 | 3 | 4 | 5 | 6 | 7 | 8 |
| 9 | 10 | 11 | 12 | 13 | 14 | 15 |
| 16 | 17 | 18 | 19 | 20 | 21 | 22 |
| 23 | 24 | 25 | 26 | 27 | 28 | 29 |
| 30 |   |   |   |   |   |   |

## december 2008

| S | M | T | W | T | F | S |
|---|---|---|---|---|---|---|
|   | 1 | 2 | 3 | 4 | 5 | 6 |
| 7 | 8 | 9 | 10 | 11 | 12 | 13 |
| 14 | 15 | 16 | 17 | 18 | 19 | 20 |
| 21 | 22 | 23 | 24 | 25 | 26 | 27 |
| 28 | 29 | 30 | 31 |   |   |   |

## january 2009

| S | M | T | W | T | F | S |
|---|---|---|---|---|---|---|
|   |   |   |   | 1 | 2 | 3 |
| 4 | 5 | 6 | 7 | 8 | 9 | 10 |
| 11 | 12 | 13 | 14 | 15 | 16 | 17 |
| 18 | 19 | 20 | 21 | 22 | 23 | 24 |
| 25 | 26 | 27 | 28 | 29 | 30 | 31 |

## february 2009

| S | M | T | W | T | F | S |
|---|---|---|---|---|---|---|
| 1 | 2 | 3 | 4 | 5 | 6 | 7 |
| 8 | 9 | 10 | 11 | 12 | 13 | 14 |
| 15 | 16 | 17 | 18 | 19 | 20 | 21 |
| 22 | 23 | 24 | 25 | 26 | 27 | 28 |

## march 2009

| S | M | T | W | T | F | S |
|---|---|---|---|---|---|---|
| 1 | 2 | 3 | 4 | 5 | 6 | 7 |
| 8 | 9 | 10 | 11 | 12 | 13 | 14 |
| 15 | 16 | 17 | 18 | 19 | 20 | 21 |
| 22 | 23 | 24 | 25 | 26 | 27 | 28 |
| 29 | 30 | 31 |   |   |   |   |

## april 2009

| S | M | T | W | T | F | S |
|---|---|---|---|---|---|---|
|   |   |   | 1 | 2 | 3 | 4 |
| 5 | 6 | 7 | 8 | 9 | 10 | 11 |
| 12 | 13 | 14 | 15 | 16 | 17 | 18 |
| 19 | 20 | 21 | 22 | 23 | 24 | 25 |
| 26 | 27 | 28 | 29 | 30 |   |   |

## may 2009

| S | M | T | W | T | F | S |
|---|---|---|---|---|---|---|
|   |   |   |   |   | 1 | 2 |
| 3 | 4 | 5 | 6 | 7 | 8 | 9 |
| 10 | 11 | 12 | 13 | 14 | 15 | 16 |
| 17 | 18 | 19 | 20 | 21 | 22 | 23 |
| 24 | 25 | 26 | 27 | 28 | 29 | 30 |
| 31 |   |   |   |   |   |   |

## june 2009

| S | M | T | W | T | F | S |
|---|---|---|---|---|---|---|
|   | 1 | 2 | 3 | 4 | 5 | 6 |
| 7 | 8 | 9 | 10 | 11 | 12 | 13 |
| 14 | 15 | 16 | 17 | 18 | 19 | 20 |
| 21 | 22 | 23 | 24 | 25 | 26 | 27 |
| 28 | 29 | 30 |   |   |   |   |

## july 2009

| S | M | T | W | T | F | S |
|---|---|---|---|---|---|---|
|   |   |   | 1 | 2 | 3 | 4 |
| 5 | 6 | 7 | 8 | 9 | 10 | 11 |
| 12 | 13 | 14 | 15 | 16 | 17 | 18 |
| 19 | 20 | 21 | 22 | 23 | 24 | 25 |
| 26 | 27 | 28 | 29 | 30 | 31 |   |

## august 2009

| S | M | T | W | T | F | S |
|---|---|---|---|---|---|---|
|   |   |   |   |   |   | 1 |
| 2 | 3 | 4 | 5 | 6 | 7 | 8 |
| 9 | 10 | 11 | 12 | 13 | 14 | 15 |
| 16 | 17 | 18 | 19 | 20 | 21 | 22 |
| 23 | 24 | 25 | 26 | 27 | 28 | 29 |
| 30 | 31 |   |   |   |   |   |

## september 2009

| S | M | T | W | T | F | S |
|---|---|---|---|---|---|---|
|   |   | 1 | 2 | 3 | 4 | 5 |
| 6 | 7 | 8 | 9 | 10 | 11 | 12 |
| 13 | 14 | 15 | 16 | 17 | 18 | 19 |
| 20 | 21 | 22 | 23 | 24 | 25 | 26 |
| 27 | 28 | 29 | 30 |   |   |   |

## october 2009

| S | M | T | W | T | F | S |
|---|---|---|---|---|---|---|
|   |   |   |   | 1 | 2 | 3 |
| 4 | 5 | 6 | 7 | 8 | 9 | 10 |
| 11 | 12 | 13 | 14 | 15 | 16 | 17 |
| 18 | 19 | 20 | 21 | 22 | 23 | 24 |
| 25 | 26 | 27 | 28 | 29 | 30 | 31 |

## november 2009

| S | M | T | W | T | F | S |
|---|---|---|---|---|---|---|
| 1 | 2 | 3 | 4 | 5 | 6 | 7 |
| 8 | 9 | 10 | 11 | 12 | 13 | 14 |
| 15 | 16 | 17 | 18 | 19 | 20 | 21 |
| 22 | 23 | 24 | 25 | 26 | 27 | 28 |
| 29 | 30 |   |   |   |   |   |

## december 2009

| S | M | T | W | T | F | S |
|---|---|---|---|---|---|---|
|   |   | 1 | 2 | 3 | 4 | 5 |
| 6 | 7 | 8 | 9 | 10 | 11 | 12 |
| 13 | 14 | 15 | 16 | 17 | 18 | 19 |
| 20 | 21 | 22 | 23 | 24 | 25 | 26 |
| 27 | 28 | 29 | 30 | 31 |   |   |

Don't miss a single day in Lean Mode.

## january 2010

| S | M | T | W | T | F | S |
|---|---|---|---|---|---|---|
|   |   |   |   |   | 1 | 2 |
| 3 | 4 | 5 | 6 | 7 | 8 | 9 |
| 10 | 11 | 12 | 13 | 14 | 15 | 16 |
| 17 | 18 | 19 | 20 | 21 | 22 | 23 |
| 24 | 25 | 26 | 27 | 28 | 29 | 30 |
| 31 |   |   |   |   |   |   |

## february 2010

| S | M | T | W | T | F | S |
|---|---|---|---|---|---|---|
|   | 1 | 2 | 3 | 4 | 5 | 6 |
| 7 | 8 | 9 | 10 | 11 | 12 | 13 |
| 14 | 15 | 16 | 17 | 18 | 19 | 20 |
| 21 | 22 | 23 | 24 | 25 | 26 | 27 |
| 28 |   |   |   |   |   |   |

## march 2010

| S | M | T | W | T | F | S |
|---|---|---|---|---|---|---|
|   | 1 | 2 | 3 | 4 | 5 | 6 |
| 7 | 8 | 9 | 10 | 11 | 12 | 13 |
| 14 | 15 | 16 | 17 | 18 | 19 | 20 |
| 21 | 22 | 23 | 24 | 25 | 26 | 27 |
| 28 | 29 | 30 | 31 |   |   |   |

## april 2010

| S | M | T | W | T | F | S |
|---|---|---|---|---|---|---|
|   |   |   |   | 1 | 2 | 3 |
| 4 | 5 | 6 | 7 | 8 | 9 | 10 |
| 11 | 12 | 13 | 14 | 15 | 16 | 17 |
| 18 | 19 | 20 | 21 | 22 | 23 | 24 |
| 25 | 26 | 27 | 28 | 29 | 30 |   |

## may 2010

| S | M | T | W | T | F | S |
|---|---|---|---|---|---|---|
|   |   |   |   |   |   | 1 |
| 2 | 3 | 4 | 5 | 6 | 7 | 8 |
| 9 | 10 | 11 | 12 | 13 | 14 | 15 |
| 16 | 17 | 18 | 19 | 20 | 21 | 22 |
| 23 | 24 | 25 | 26 | 27 | 28 | 29 |
| 30 | 31 |   |   |   |   |   |

## june 2010

| S | M | T | W | T | F | S |
|---|---|---|---|---|---|---|
|   |   | 1 | 2 | 3 | 4 | 5 |
| 6 | 7 | 8 | 9 | 10 | 11 | 12 |
| 13 | 14 | 15 | 16 | 17 | 18 | 19 |
| 20 | 21 | 22 | 23 | 24 | 25 | 26 |
| 27 | 28 | 29 | 30 |   |   |   |

## july 2010

| S | M | T | W | T | F | S |
|---|---|---|---|---|---|---|
|   |   |   |   | 1 | 2 | 3 |
| 4 | 5 | 6 | 7 | 8 | 9 | 10 |
| 11 | 12 | 13 | 14 | 15 | 16 | 17 |
| 18 | 19 | 20 | 21 | 22 | 23 | 24 |
| 25 | 26 | 27 | 28 | 29 | 30 | 31 |

## august 2010

| S | M | T | W | T | F | S |
|---|---|---|---|---|---|---|
| 1 | 2 | 3 | 4 | 5 | 6 | 7 |
| 8 | 9 | 10 | 11 | 12 | 13 | 14 |
| 15 | 16 | 17 | 18 | 19 | 20 | 21 |
| 22 | 23 | 24 | 25 | 26 | 27 | 28 |
| 29 | 30 | 31 |   |   |   |   |

## september 2010

| S | M | T | W | T | F | S |
|---|---|---|---|---|---|---|
|   |   |   | 1 | 2 | 3 | 4 |
| 5 | 6 | 7 | 8 | 9 | 10 | 11 |
| 12 | 13 | 14 | 15 | 16 | 17 | 18 |
| 19 | 20 | 21 | 22 | 23 | 24 | 25 |
| 26 | 27 | 28 | 29 | 30 |   |   |

## october 2010

| S | M | T | W | T | F | S |
|---|---|---|---|---|---|---|
|   |   |   |   |   | 1 | 2 |
| 3 | 4 | 5 | 6 | 7 | 8 | 9 |
| 10 | 11 | 12 | 13 | 14 | 15 | 16 |
| 17 | 18 | 19 | 20 | 21 | 22 | 23 |
| 24 | 25 | 26 | 27 | 28 | 29 | 30 |
| 31 |   |   |   |   |   |   |

## november 2010

| S | M | T | W | T | F | S |
|---|---|---|---|---|---|---|
|   | 1 | 2 | 3 | 4 | 5 | 6 |
| 7 | 8 | 9 | 10 | 11 | 12 | 13 |
| 14 | 15 | 16 | 17 | 18 | 19 | 20 |
| 21 | 22 | 23 | 24 | 25 | 26 | 27 |
| 28 | 29 | 30 |   |   |   |   |

## december 2010

| S | M | T | W | T | F | S |
|---|---|---|---|---|---|---|
|   |   |   | 1 | 2 | 3 | 4 |
| 5 | 6 | 7 | 8 | 9 | 10 | 11 |
| 12 | 13 | 14 | 15 | 16 | 17 | 18 |
| 19 | 20 | 21 | 22 | 23 | 24 | 25 |
| 26 | 27 | 28 | 29 | 30 | 31 |   |

## january 2011

| S | M | T | W | T | F | S |
|---|---|---|---|---|---|---|
|   |   |   |   |   |   | 1 |
| 2 | 3 | 4 | 5 | 6 | 7 | 8 |
| 9 | 10 | 11 | 12 | 13 | 14 | 15 |
| 16 | 17 | 18 | 19 | 20 | 21 | 22 |
| 23 | 24 | 25 | 26 | 27 | 28 | 29 |
| 30 | 31 |   |   |   |   |   |

## february 2011

| S | M | T | W | T | F | S |
|---|---|---|---|---|---|---|
|   |   | 1 | 2 | 3 | 4 | 5 |
| 6 | 7 | 8 | 9 | 10 | 11 | 12 |
| 13 | 14 | 15 | 16 | 17 | 18 | 19 |
| 20 | 21 | 22 | 23 | 24 | 25 | 26 |
| 27 | 28 |   |   |   |   |   |

## march 2011

| S | M | T | W | T | F | S |
|---|---|---|---|---|---|---|
|   |   | 1 | 2 | 3 | 4 | 5 |
| 6 | 7 | 8 | 9 | 10 | 11 | 12 |
| 13 | 14 | 15 | 16 | 17 | 18 | 19 |
| 20 | 21 | 22 | 23 | 24 | 25 | 26 |
| 27 | 28 | 29 | 30 | 31 |   |   |